Drugs Handbook 1986–7

Drugs Handbook 1986-7

Paul Turner

Professor of Clinical Pharmacology, St Bartholomew's Hospital, London EC1

and

Glyn N. Volans

Consultant Clinical Pharmacologist and Director of the Poisons Unit, Guy's Hospital, London SE1

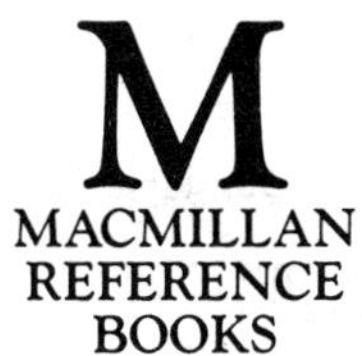

MACMILLAN
REFERENCE
BOOKS

Sixth revised edition published 1986 by
THE MACMILLAN PRESS LTD
London and Basingstoke

Associated Companies in Auckland, Delhi, Dublin, Gaborone, Hamburg, Harare, Hong Kong, Johannesburg, Kuala Lumpur, Lagos, Manzini, Melbourne, Mexico City, Nairobi, New York, Singapore, Tokyo.

British Library Cataloguing in Publication Data

Drugs handbook.—1987
1. Drugs—Catalogs
I. Turner, Paul, *1933-* II. Volans, Glyn
615′.1′0941 RS355

ISBN 0–333–41815–8
ISSN 0265–3931

Typeset by
MB Graphics (Typesetting) Services, Dunstable, Bedfordshire

Printed and bound in Great Britain by
Anchor Brendon Ltd, Tiptree, Essex

Contents

PREFACE

This revised edition contains new products introduced during the last year and has been fully revised to take account of withdrawals and revisions. We have considered taking account of the so-called limited list but think that it cannot be accomodated directly in this text in view of the number and frequency of the revisions to the list. For further information on this list the reader is referred to the relevant section in the Introduction.

May 1986

PAUL TURNER
GLYN N. VOLANS

INTRODUCTION

Patient care has now extended far beyond the patient–doctor relationship and involves several different highly trained health care professions, including amongst others nurses, midwives, occupational therapists, physiotherapists, radiographers, electro-encephalographers, dieticians, social workers, psychologists and medical secretaries. Although prescribing of medicines is the responsibility of a doctor, the drugs which medicines contain may influence patients in many ways, and it is important that others involved in a patient's health care should have ready access to information on the various medicines which he or she may receive, either by prescription or by over-the-counter purchase. The primary purpose of this book is to provide such information for these and other groups within the health professions. It is not a textbook of clinical pharmacology or medical treatment nor is it intended to be: rather it is meant to be a short guide to the mechanism of action, therapeutic indications and chief unwanted effects of most medicines available in the United Kingdom.

Drugs and Medicines

A doctor usually prescribes a *drug*, but the patient receives a *medicine*. The medicine is the whole formulation in which the drug, that is the active substance, is combined with other ingredients to form a convenient form of administration, such as a tablet, capsule, suppository, inhalation, ointment or injection. We have not included all constituents of the medicines listed in this book, but have mentioned only those substances which we believe may contribute to the therapeutic or adverse effects of the medicine involved. It must be stressed that the mention of a medicine in this book, and statements about its indications, do not imply that it is necessarily an effective treatment, or that the authors believe it to be such; in fact we believe that for large numbers of drugs there is no good evidence of their effectiveness.

Names of Drugs

Most drugs have at least three names. The first is the full chemical name, which is too long and complicated to use regularly. More convenient is the shorter *generic* or *approved* name, which may become accepted internationally. Finally, there is the *brand* or *trade* name, given by the pharmaceutical manufacturer for its own particular brand or formulation. For example, 4-amino-5-chloro-*N*-(2-diethylaminoethyl)-2-methoxybenzamide hydrochloride is the chemical name for metoclopramide hydrochloride, the approved name of the drug marketed at present by at least two drug firms under the brand names Maxolon and Primperan. We have distinguished between approved and brand names by compiling two separate alphabetical lists. The main body of the book is devoted to approved names, with a brand name index at the end, and to save space and avoid duplication of information almost all the brand names have been cross-referenced to the appropriate approved names. Also in the interests of saving space, where a number of drugs have essentially similar effects we have cross-referenced approved names to those which we consider to be the most typical and most frequently prescribed. Thus all cross-references refer to the list of approved names, and are shown in bold type, for example, **Amethocaine**.

Drugs in Pregnancy

Several drugs are known to be hazardous to the developing foetus and for most drugs there is no definite information on their safety in pregnancy. We have avoided constant repetition of this but would stress that in pregnancy all drugs should be used with caution and only when essential.

Drug Combinations

Many of the preparations listed in this book are combinations of drugs rather than individual ones. The majority are rather crude attempts at what might be called 'blunderbuss treatment' of a variety of signs and symptoms, but some have been developed on scientific grounds to exploit the interaction of two or more drugs working together. Others, by combining drugs that are commonly used together, offer, if correctly used, a means of simplifying treatment for patients on long-term multiple drugs and thus improve compliance, for example, combination drugs for hypertension. Attempts have been made to coin suitable names for such combinations, for example co-trimazine, co-trimoxazole, but this has not proved generally possible and so it is becoming accepted practice to prescribe such preparations, like most other combination products, by their trade names.

Limited list

In 1985 the government issued a 'black list' of drugs and preparations that cannot be prescribed or dispensed under the NHS but only on private prescriptions, the patient having to pay for them in full. These restrictions on prescribing and dispensing at the public expense are at present limited to the following therapeutic groups:

- Antacids
- Laxatives
- Analgesics used for mild or moderate pain
- Cough and cold remedies, which include cough suppressants, expectorants, mucolytics, inhalations, and nasal decongestants
- Tonics
- Vitamins
- Benzodiazpine tranquillizers, sedatives and hypnotics

An advisory committee has been set up to advise the DHSS on changes that should be made in the list. Doctors and pharmacists are able to recognize which drugs and medicines cannot be prescribed under the NHS by a symbol published against their names in the *British National Formulary.*

Technical Terms, Further Information

This book has not been written for the general public, and it assumes a basic knowledge and understanding of human biology and disease. Many readers may, nevertheless, wish to refer to larger books for more complete and detailed information, and we would recommend:

1. For information on drugs:
   Turner, P., Richens, A. and Routledge, P. *Clinical Pharmacology.* 5th Edition, 1986. Churchill–Livingstone, London.
   Laurence, D. R. and Bennett, P. N. *Clinical Pharmacology.* 5th Edition. 1980. Churchill–Livingstone, London.
   Goodman, L. S. and Gilman, A. (Eds.) *The Pharmacological Basis of Therapeutics.* 7th Edition, 1985. Baillière Tindall, London.
   Reynolds, J. E. F. (Ed.) Martindale: *The Extra Pharmocopoeia.* 28th Edition, 1982. Pharmaceutical Press, London.
2. For information on diseases and their management:
   Houston, J. C., Joiner, C. L. and Trounce, J. R. *A Short Textbook of Medicine.* 7th Edition, 1982. Hodder and Stoughton, London.
   Mann, W. N. (Ed.) Conybeare's *Textbook of Medicine.* 16th Edition, 1975. Churchill–Livingstone, London.
3. For information on treatment of poisoning:
   Henry, J. and Volans, G. *ABC of Poisoning. Part I: Drugs.* 1984 British Medical Journal, London.

March 1986

PAUL TURNER
GLYN N. VOLANS

ACKNOWLEDGEMENTS

The authors would like to express their thanks and gratitude to Hazel Boughton for her help in compiling the lists of drugs and for typing the manuscript.

ABBREVIATIONS

The following abbreviations have been used throughout the book:

(b) indicates a borderline substance, that is a substance which may only be prescribed as a drug under certain conditions.

(c) indicates a drug whose prescription is controlled under the Misuse of Drugs Act.

(d) discontinued by the manufacturers during the year prior to publication. As supplies will still be available from pharmacies until stocks run out, these products have not yet been deleted from our lists.

CNS Central nervous system.

DEFINITIONS OF DRUG GROUP NAMES AND MEDICAL TERMS

abortifacient Used to produce abortion.

adjuvant Something added to a drug which aids or modifies the main ingredient.

adrenergic Has similar actions to adrenaline.

agonist Has an observable effect within the body, resulting from a direct action upon a specific receptor.

aminoglycoside Drug with a chemical structure related to **Streptomycin**.

anabolic Stimulates cell metabolism causing increased tissue growth.

analgesic Relieves pain.

anorectic Appetite suppressant used in obesity.

antacid Neutralizes acid produced by the stomach.

antagonist Opposes the action or blocks the effect of another drug.

anticholinergic Blocks the action of **Acetylcholine** or cholinergic (acetylcholine-like) drugs.

anticholinesterase Blocks the action of cholinesterase–a naturally occurring enzyme which breaks down **Acetylcholine** bringing its action to an end. The effect of the anticholinesterase is therefore to prolong and intensify the action of acetylcholine.

anticoagulant Prevents blood from clotting.

anticonvulsant Stops or prevents epileptic seizures.

antiemetic Prevents nausea and vomiting.

antihypertensive Lowers blood pressure.

antipyretic Lowers body temperature in febrile conditions.

antiserotonin Blocks the action of serotonin.

antispasmodic Relieves spasm of muscles, for example, in the gastro-intestinal tract (gastro-intestinal colic).

antitussive Suppresses cough.

anxiolytic Reduces anxiety.

arrhythmia Disorder of rhythm, generally of the heart.

astringent Precipitates protein to form a protective layer over damaged skin or mucous membranes.

bactericidal Kills bacteria.

bacteriostatic Inhibits growth of bacteria but does not kill them.

bioavailability Extent to which and rate at which the active substance in a drug is taken up by the body in a form that is physiologically active.

bradycardia Slow heart rate.

bronchodilator Increases the diameter of the airways in the respiratory system and thus reduces the physical resistance to breathing.

buffer Solution that opposes changes in acidity or alkalinity.

cardioselective Acts on the heart without the other effects usually found in drugs of a particular group, for example beta-adrenoceptor blocking drugs. In practice, the cardioselectivity is usually relative and the other effects can be traced, although in a less pronounced form.

carminative Facilitates the eructation of gas from the stomach.

cathartic   Relieves constipation.
cholinergic   Has actions similar to **Acetylcholine**.
corticosteroids   Hormones (natural or synthetic) with actions on metabolism and against tissue inflammation. The natural hormones are produced by the adrenal gland.
cycloplegic   Paralyzes muscle of the eye controlling accommodation. Leads to blurred vision.
cytotoxic   Has toxic effects upon living cells which reduce growth or cause destruction of the cells.
decongestant   Reduces congestion (i.e. swelling) of the nasal mucosa.
demulcent   Supposed to coat and smooth mucous membranes of the gastro-intestinal tract (e.g., milk, raw egg white).
diuretic   Increases urine output.
elixir   Clear, flavoured liquid preparation of drug frequently containing alcohol and sweetening and colouring agents.
emetic   Induces vomiting.
enema   Drug formulation for rectal administration.
enteric coating   Surface coating of capsules or tablets designed to resist gastric acid acting on it, so that the drug is not released until reaching the small intestine.
expectorant   Aids removal of sputum from the lungs and respiratory passages.
fibrinolytic   Dissolves or otherwise destroys the fibrin which is formed when blood clots.
G6PD   Glucose 6-phosphate dehydrogenase: an enzyme involved in carbohydrate metabolism. Some patients exhibit an inherited deficiency of this enzyme and are thus more susceptible to certain diseases and adverse drug effects.
haematinic   Involved in the normal development of red blood cells.
haemostatic   Stops bleeding and prevents blood loss.
herbicide   Kills plants.
hormone   Naturally occurring substance which is secreted by a gland into the blood stream, whence it is carried to the part of the body on which it acts. Insulin, for example, is secreted by the pancreas and acts at sites all over the body.
hypotensive   Lowers blood pressure.
hypnotic   Facilitates sleep.
hypoglycaemic   Lowers the blood glucose.
immunosuppressant   Tends to suppress the immune response. This effect may be used to suppress some cancers or rejection of transplanted organs, but makes the body more susceptible to infections.
infusion   Administration of a drug by continuous intravenous drip/injection.
insecticide   Kills insects.

laxative Relieves constipation.

linctus Viscous liquid preparation of drug containing sugar or alternative sweetening agent.

lotion Wet dressing used to cleanse and cool inflammed skin lesions.

melaena Black stools due to passage of altered blood from haemorrhage.

miotic Constricts pupil of the eye.

mucolytic Liquifies mucus within the respiratory system.

mydriatic Dilates the pupil of the eye.

narcotic analgesic Pain-relieving drug of the opium group. Liable to have addictive properties.

nephrotoxic Causes damage to the kidneys.

neurotransmitter Biochemical substance which acts in the transmission of nerve impulses.

ototoxic Causes damage to nerves involved in hearing.

parasympathomimetic Has actions similar to the parasympathetic chemical transmitter in the nervous system **Acetylcholine**.

parenteral Administered by a route other than via the gastro-intestinal tract. Usually refers to intradermal, subcutaneous, intramuscular or intravenous injection.

pessary Solid-dose drug formulation similar to suppository but placed in the vagina. Usually used for local actions in the vagina but systemic absorption of the drug may occur.

pesticide Kills pests. This term includes a wide range of compounds (e.g., rodenticides which kill rats and small mammals, insecticides, herbicides). Only a few of these chemicals also have applications as drugs.

pharmacodynamics Study of the actions of drugs in living systems.

pharmacokinetics Study of the fate of drugs in the body. Includes absorption, distribution, metabolism and excretion.

phenothiazine Drug with a chemical structure similar to **Chlorpromazine**.

placebo Inactive substance or preparation used in controlled studies to evaluate the effectiveness of a medicinal substance. In some instances, a placebo may be prescribed to satisfy the patient's desire for medicine. In other instances, a supposedly 'active' drug may be prescribed but the benefits seen relate not to this action but to the 'placebo' effect.

prophylactic Tends to prevent a condition rather than treat it when established.

purgative Facilitates evacuation of the bowels.

receptor Site on cell surfaces which reacts to drugs or endogenous substance to produce the observed effect.

rubefacient Causes reddening of the skin.

sedative Reduces arousal.

suppository Solid-dose, elongated, cone-shaped drug formulation for insertion into the rectum for local treatment (e.g., for haemorrhoids) or for drug absorption (e.g., anti-emetic). Has a fatty base which melts at body temperature.

sustained-release formulation   Product specifically designed to release the active drug more slowly and over a prolonged period. Used to reduce the interval between doses and to prevent toxicity from high drug concentrations achieved in the body when there is rapid absorption.

sympathomimetic   Has actions similar to the chemical transmitters of sympathetic nervous system (**Adrenaline** and **Noradrenaline**).

tachycardia   Rapid heart rate.

tachyphylaxis   Occurs when repeated doses of the drug produce progressively smaller effects (or else progressively bigger doses are required).

teratogenic   May produce congenital malformation if given during the first three months of pregnancy.

thiazide   Drug with a chemical structure similar to **Chlorothiazide**.

topical   Applied externally at the site where the drug action is needed (e.g., for treatment of skin rashes or eye infections).

toxoid   A preparation of a bacterial toxin that has its toxic properties removed but has retained its ability to stimulate the body's immunity to it by the production of antibodies.

tranquillizer   Drug with sedative actions on the brain which is used in the treatment and management of certain psychiatric disorders, for example, schizophrenia, mania.

vaccine   Preparation of live attenuated or dead microorganisms used to induce immunity.

vasoconstrictor   Causes constriction of blood vessels.

vasodilator   Causes dilatation of blood vessels.

vitamin   Chemical essential in small amounts for maintenance of normal growth and health. Must be obtained from external sources usually dietary. Inadequate intake leads to deficiency diseases.

Part I

Approved Names

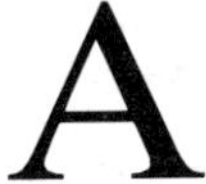

Acebutolol Beta-adrenoceptor blocking drug, with limited cardioselectivity. Uses, side effects, etc. as for **Propranolol**.

Acetaminophen USA: see **Paracetamol**.

Acetazolamide Weak diuretic. Also used in glaucoma to reduce intraocular pressure, and as an anticonvulsant. Acts by inhibiting carbonic anhydrase and so reduces hydrogen ions available for exchange with sodium ions. May cause drowsiness, mental confusion, and paraesthesia.

Acetohexamide Oral antidiabetic agent with actions and uses similar to **Chlorpropamide**.

Acetomenaphthone See **Vitamin K**.

Acetylcholine Neurotransmitter, particularly in parasympathetic system. Peripheral effects include miosis, paralysis of accommodation, increased glandular secretions, contraction of smooth muscle in gastro-intestinal, respiratory and urogenital systems, slowing of heart, and vasodilation. These effects blocked by **Atropine sulphate**. Not used clinically.

Acetylcysteine Mucolytic. Administered by mouth or by inhalation from a nebulizer. Liquefies mucus and aids expectoration in diseases where mucus is troublesome (e.g., chronic bronchitis). May cause bronchospasm, haemoptysis, nausea, and vomiting. Used also in lubricant eye drops and intravenously in the treatment of **Paracetamol** overdosage where it prevents liver damage by restoring or acting as a substitute for depleted liver glutathione stores. In this use may also cause rash, nausea, vomiting, and transient bronchospasm.

Acetylsalicylic acid (Aspirin) Anti-inflammatory, antipyretic analgesic. Inhibits prostaglandin synthesis, reduces stickiness of blood platelets. May cause gastric erosion and haemorrhage, hypersensitivity reactions. Tinnitus and hyperventilation leading to respiratory and cardiovascular failure in overdose. Interacts with oral anticoagulants and sulphonylureas. Forced alkaline diuresis may be used to speed elimination in overdosage.

Acrosoxacin Antibiotic used only in treatment of gonorrhoea where the patient is allergic to **Penicillin** or organism is resistant to penicillins and other antibiotics. Needs only single dose. May cause dizziness, drowsiness, headache, and gastro-intestinal disturbances.

Actinomycin D Cytotoxic antibiotic used in neoplastic disease. Adverse effects include bone marrow depression.

Activated charcoal Charcoal is a strong adsorbant. 'Activated' indicates simply that the charcoal meets certain standards in adsorbence tests. Used by mouth in cases of acute poisoning to reduce absorption of drugs or other toxins. May cause nausea and vomiting. Would adsorb oral emetics or antidotes and therefore not used if these are given. Subsequent black stools should not be mistaken for melaena.

Acyclovir Antiviral agent used orally, topically and intravenously to treat herpes simplex infections. Should not be used when patient is dehydrated as may cause rise in blood urea and creatinine.

Adenosine monophosphoric acid (AMP) Source of high-energy phosphate bonds for tissue metabolism. Suggested for use in cardiovascular disease and rheumatism but efficacy unproven.

Adenosine triphosphoric acid (ATP) Source of high-energy phosphate bonds for tissue metabolism. Suggested for use in cardiovascular disease and rheumatism but efficacy unproven.

Adrenaline Sympathomimetic amine, alpha and beta-adrenoceptor agonist. Produces vasoconstriction with rise in blood pressure, cardio-acceleration and bronchodilation. Used in acute allergic reactions, as peripheral vasoconstrictor in narrow-angle glaucoma and in cardiac arrest. Toxicity includes hypertension, pulmonary oedema, and cardiac arrhythmias.

Agar Purgative. Increases faecal bulk by same mechanism as **Methylcellulose** but less effective.

Alclofenac Anti-inflammatory analgesic with actions similar to **Ibuprofen**.

Alcuronium Skeletal muscle relaxant with uses and adverse effects similar to **Tubocurarine**.

Aldosterone Naturally occurring adrenal (mineralocorticoid) steroid hormone. Acts mainly on salt and water metabolism by increasing salt retention in the kidney; has no useful anti-inflammatory activity. Used only in replacement therapy for adrenal insufficiency.

Alexitol sodium Complex of sodium poly(hydroxyaluminium) carbonate and hexitol. An antacid with uses and adverse effects similar to **Aluminium hydroxide**.

Alfentanil (c) Narcotic analgesic, with actions and uses similar to **Fentanyl** and **Morphine**. Has a rapid onset of action, but its duration of action is less than other narcotic analgesics. Used as an adjunct to anaesthesia during short surgical procedures.

Alginic acid Extract of algae found mainly on the west coast of Scotland and Ireland. Used as tablet binder and disintegrant.

Allantoin Used in creams and lotions to stimulate wound healing.

Allergen extract vaccines Extracts prepared from common allergens (e.g., grass, bee venom) for hyposensitization of hypersensitive individuals. Used as graded doses starting from the lowest. Injected subcutaneously. Avoid in pregnancy, febrile conditions and acute asthma. May cause allergic reactions.

Allopurinol Reduces formation of uric acid from purine precursors by inhibiting the enzyme xanthine oxidase. Used in primary and secondary gout.

Allyloestrenol Hormone with actions similar to **Progesterone**.

Almasilate Polymer of aluminium magnesium silicate. Similar antacid properties to **Aluminium hydroxide** and **Magnesium trisilicate**.

Aloes Derived from species of aloe. Used as purgative, producing motion six to twelve hours after ingestion. Causes griping. Colours urine red. May cause nephritis in large doses.

Aloin Extract of aloes: see **Aloes**.

Aloxiprin Complex of **Aluminium antacids** and **Acetylsalicylic acid**, yielding these agents after breakdown in the gastro-intestinal tract.

Alpha-calcidol (1 α-Hydroxyvitamin D_3) Rapidly converted in the liver to dihydroxyvitamin D_3–the metabolite of vitamin D with the most marked effect on calcium and phosphate balance. Used in treatment of renal bone disease, hypoparathyroidism, rickets, and osteomalacia when these are resistant to vitamin D itself. May cause hypercalcaemia with risk of metastatic calcification and renal failure. Hypercalcaemia treated by stopping the drug and administration of fluids plus potent diuretics (e.g., **Frusemide**).

Alphadolone See **Alphaxalone**.

Alphaxalone Steroid used as intravenous anaesthetic, in combination with **Alphadolone**.

Alprazolam Benzodiazepine anxiolytic, with actions and adverse effects similar to **Diazepam**. May also have antidepressant effects. Used for short-term treatment of anxiety and anxiety associated with depression.

Alprenolol Beta-adrenoceptor blocking drug with partial agonist activity (intrinsic sympathomimetic activity). Uses, side effects, etc. as for **Propranolol**.

Alprostadil (Prostaglandin E_1) Used to maintain foetal cardiac circulation prior to corrective surgery in neonates with congenital heart abnormalities.

Alum (Potassium aluminium sulphate) Used as solid to stop bleeding; in powder for application to umbilical cord. Precipitates proteins and is a powerful astringent.

Aluminium antacids Range of aluminium salts, used alone or complexed with other compounds. Neutralize gastric acid in treatment of peptic ulceration. Large doses cause constipation which may be prevented by combination with **Magnesium antacids**. May reduce absorption of other drugs (e.g., **Tetracycline**).

Aluminium carbonate Nonsystemic (nonabsorbable) antacid. Used in treatment of peptic ulceration where it produces longer neutralization of acid than **Sodium bicarbonate**. Also used in prevention of urinary phosphate stones. May cause constipation. Reduces absorption of **Tetracycline** given at same time.

Aluminium chloride Astringent. Precipitates proteins when applied to skin resulting in hardening and reduced secretions. Used to prevent excessive sweating (hyperhidrosis).

Aluminium chlorohydrate Used topically in antiperspirant preparations.

Aluminium glycinate See **Aluminium antacids**.

Aluminium hydroxide Nonsystemic (nonabsorbable) antacid. Neutralizes gastric acid and binds phosphate ions in the gut. Used to treat peptic ulceration by reducing gastric acidity and also to increase phosphate excretion when phosphate retention is associated with stone formation (e.g., renal stones). Large doses cause constipation which may be prevented by combination with **Magnesium antacids**.

Alverine Antispasmodic drug used in gut colic; related to **Papaverine**.

Amantadine Antiviral agent for prophylaxis against influenza. Antiparkinsonian drug used in mild cases. Adverse effects include dry mouth, visual disturbance, confusion, hallucinations, and ankle oedema.

Ambenonium Anticholinesterase: similar to **Pyridostigmine**.

Ambucetamide Antispasmodic used in preparations recommended for dysmenorrhoea.

Ambutonium Anticholinergic with actions similar to **Atropine sulphate**. Used in treatment of peptic ulcer.

Amethocaine Local anaesthetic similar to **Lignocaine**. Powerful surface activity but toxic by injection. Used topically in ophthalmology.

Amikacin Antimicrobial with actions and uses similar to **Gentamicin**.

Amiloride Potassium-sparing diuretic. Acts by inhibiting exchange of sodium for potassium in the distal tubule of the kidney. Relatively weak diuretic used when there is particular danger of potassium loss (e.g., fluid overload due to liver failure). Often combined with a thiazide (e.g., **Bendrofluazide**) or **Frusemide**. Danger of excessive potassium retention. May cause nausea, vomiting and diarrhoea.

Aminacrine Skin disinfectant.

Amino acids Dietary components. Breakdown products of proteins. Some may be synthesized in the body, others (the 'essential' amino acids) cannot, and must be taken in at least minimum amounts for normal health.

Aminoacridine See **Aminacrine**.

Aminobenzoic acid Member of the vitamin B complex found in some compound vitamin preparations. Used as a lotion to protect the skin from ultraviolet radiation.

Aminocaproic acid See **Epsilon-aminocaproic acid**.

Aminoglutethimide Analogue of the hypnotic **Glutethimide** originally used as an anticonvulsant. Has inhibitory actions on adrenal cortex. May be used to suppress adrenal activity in hyperadrenalism, particularly when due to adrenal carcinoma. Also used to reduce oedema caused by hyperaldosteronism and in prostatic carcinoma. Adverse effects include drowsiness, confusion, skin rashes, gastric discomfort, bone marrow suppression, hypothyroidism, and virilism.

Aminophylline (Theophylline ethylenediamine) Relaxes smooth muscle, dilates bronchi, increases heart rate and force, and has diuretic action. Used in cardiac and bronchial asthma. Given orally, intravenously, or by suppository. Adverse effects include nausea, vomiting, if given orally; vertigo, restlessness, cardiac arrhythmias, if given intravenously.

5-Aminosalicylic acid See **Mesalazine**.

Amiodarone Cardiac antiarrhythmic. Adverse effects include hepatitis, disturbances of thyroid function, corneal deposits, nerve damage, skin photosensitivity, sleep disturbance, and a metallic taste.

Amitriptyline Antidepressant. Actions and adverse effects similar to **Imipramine**. Also has sedative and anxiolytic properties.

Ammonium chloride Acidifying agent. Also used as expectorant and diuretic.

Amodiaquine Antimalarial with actions and uses similar to **Chloroquine**. Generally well tolerated, but may cause nausea, vomiting, diarrhoea, and lethargy. Long-term use may lead to corneal deposits and bluish discolouration of nails, skin, and hard palate–clears slowly when treatment stopped.

Amoxycillin Similar to **Ampicillin** but better absorbed.

Amphetamine (c) Sympathomimetic amine. Increases heart rate and blood pressure by **Noradrenaline** release from sympathetic nerve endings. Produces central stimulation through central noradrenergic and dopaminergic receptor activity. Many uses including as anorectic. Produces dependence and, in prolonged, excessive use, psychosis. Now falling into disuse.

Amphotericin B Antifungal. Used topically for skin infections or by intravenous injection for severe generalized fungal infections. Topically it may produce irritation of skin. Systemic side effects are often severe, including headache, vomiting, fever, joint pains, convulsions, and kidney damage.

Ampicillin Penicillin antibiotic with broader spectrum of activity than benzylpenicillin; active against typhoid fever. Adverse effects as for **Benzylpenicillin**. Rash common if given to patients with infectious mononucleosis (i.e. glandular fever).

Amsacrine Cytotoxic drug with actions, indications and adverse effects similar to **Doxorubicin**.

Amylobarbitone (c) Barbiturate hypnotic/sedative. General depressant action on CNS. Used in treatment of insomnia and anxiety. Frequently has a 'hangover' effect with impairment of mental and physical performance. Tolerance and addiction may occur, with insomnia, delirium and convulsions on withdrawal. Metabolized by liver and therefore used with caution in liver disease. Induces its own metabolism and that of some other drugs with danger of adverse drug interaction. Coma with respiratory depression in overdosage. No antidote; treated by supportive measures.

Amylocaine Local anaesthetic with actions similar to **Lignocaine**.

Ancrod Anticoagulant enzyme from venom of Malayan Pit Viper. Given intravenously. May produce allergic reactions.

Anethole Essential oil with odour of anise. Used as a carminative and expectorant.

Aneurine (Thiamine, Vitamin B_1) Vitamin. Deficiency may cause cardiac failure (wet beri-beri), peripheral neuritis (dry beri-beri) and Wernicke's encephalopathy.

Angiotensin Peptide pressor agent given by intravenous infusion in treatment of hypotensive states and shock. Adverse effects include headache and cardiac arrhythmias.

Antazoline Antihistamine with actions and uses similar to **Promethazine**.

Anthroquinone glycosides Derivative of Chinese rhubarb used with **Salicylic acid** for topical treatment of inflammed and ulcerated conditions in the mouth.

Antidiuretic hormone See **Vasopressin**.

Aprotinin Inhibits enzymes that digest proteins. Used in acute pancreatitis. Adverse effects include allergic reactions.

Arginine Essential amino acid used in treatment of liver coma and in tests of growth hormone secretion.

Ascorbic acid See **Vitamin C**.

Aspirin See **Acetylsalicylic acid**.

Astemizole Antihistamine with actions and adverse effects similar to **Terfenadine**.

Atenolol Beta-adrenoceptor blocking drug with limited cardioselectivity. Uses, side effects, etc. as for **Propranolol**.

Atracurium Skeletal muscle relaxant with uses and adverse effects similar to **Tubocurarine**.

Atropine See **Atropine sulphate**.

Atropine methonitrate Anticholinergic with actions, uses, and adverse effects similar to **Atropine sulphate**, but has less effects upon CNS and is sometimes considered less toxic.

Atropine sulphate Parasympatholytic derivative of belladonna plants (e.g., deadly nightshade). Blocks peripheral autonomic cholinergic nerve junctions. Causes dilatation of pupils, paralysis of ocular accommodation, tachycardia, reduced gut motility, decreased secretions, and CNS stimulation. Used intravenously in treatment of bradycardia and anticholinesterase poisoning (e.g., due to organophosphorus insecticides), intramuscularly as part of pre-operative medication, and topically in the eye for optical refraction in children. For parkinsonism and peptic ulceration it has largely been replaced by other anticholinergics. May cause dry mouth, blurred vision, glaucoma, and retention of urine. In overdosage, there is tachycardia, fever, flushed skin, dehydration and excitement. Anticholinesterase (e.g., **Neostigmine**) may be used as antidote.

Attapulgite Form of magnesium aluminium silicate used as absorbent and adsorbent agent in treatment of acute poisoning, in diarrhoea and in topical deodorant preparations.

Aurothiomalate sodium Preparation of gold for intramuscular injection in treatment of active rheumatoid arthritis. Adverse effects include allergic reactions such as rashes, blood dyscrasias, jaundice, kidney dysfunction, peripheral neuritis, and encephalitis.

Azapropazone Non-steroid anti-inflammatory/analgesic used in arthritic conditions. Adverse effects include some gastro-intestinal disturbances, although not as often as with **Acetylsalicylic acid**, and allergic rashes.

Azatadine Antihistamine with actions, uses, and adverse effects similar to **Promethazine**.

Azathioprine Derivative of **Mercaptopurine**, used primarily as immunosuppressant agent in patients receiving organ transplants. Adverse effects include bone marrow depression.

Azlocillin Broad-spectrum antibiotic, with actions and adverse effects similar to **Carbenicillin**.

B

Bacampicillin Prodrug antibiotic. Readily absorbed from gastro-intestinal tract and rapidly metabolized to the active drug **Ampicillin**, whose actions, uses, and adverse effects it shares.

Bacitracin Peptide antibiotic active mainly on gram-positive cocci. Nephrotoxic on systemic administration. Only used topically for skin infections.

Baclofen Used in treatment of skeletal muscle spasticity. Adverse effects include nausea and sedation.

Bamethan Vasodilator with actions and adverse effects similar to **Tolazoline**.

Beclamide Anticonvulsant drug that is claimed to possess stimulant rather than sedative properties.

Beclomethasone Potent synthetic **Corticosteroid** similar to **Dexamethasone**. Used by inhalation for treatment of asthma.

Belladonna extract Plant extract containing **Atropine sulphate** and having similar actions, uses, and adverse effects.

Bendrofluazide Thiazide diuretic used in the treatment of fluid overload and in control of high blood pressure. Acts by reducing sodium reabsorption in the kidney. Less potent than **Frusemide** and **Mersalyl** but has longer action. It is effective orally. May cause excessive loss of potassium in urine and increase in blood uric acid or glucose. Consequently can produce symptoms of hypokalaemia, gout, or diabetes. May produce impotence.

Benethamine penicillin Long-acting form of **Benzylpenicillin**, with similar actions and adverse effects.

Benorylate Analgesic/anti-inflammatory combination that breaks down in the body into **Acetylsalicylic acid** and **Paracetamol**, and has the actions of each.

Benoxaprofen Non-steroid anti-inflammatory/analgesic with actions and uses similar to **Ibuprofen**. Adverse effects include photosensitive skin rashes, gastro-intestinal irritation, and liver damage. Withdrawn from use in 1982.

Benoxinate See **Oxibuprocaine**.

Benperidol Tranquillizer, with actions, uses, etc. similar to **Haloperidol**.

Benserazide Used with **Levodopa** in Parkinson's disease. Prevents peripheral breakdown of **Levodopa**, allowing reduced dosage and decreased side effects.

Bentonite Native colloidal hydrated aluminium silicate used as an absorbant in treatment of poisoning, and as a pharmaceutical aid in preparation of drug formulations.

Benzalkonium Topical disinfectant used in creams, lozenges, and irrigating solutions.

Benzamine Local anaesthetic with actions similar to **Lignocaine**.

Benzathine penicillin Long-acting form of **Benzylpenicillin**, with similar actions and adverse effects.

Benzethonium Similar to **Benzalkonium**.

Benzhexol Antispasmodic parasympatholytic used in parkinsonism of all causes. Like **Atropine**, it may produce dry mouth, blurred vision, constipation, hesitancy of micturition, confusion, and hallucinations. Contra-indicated in glaucoma and prostate hypertrophy. In overdosage, dry mouth, nausea, vomiting, excitement, confusion, hot dry skin, rapid pulse, and fixed dilated pupils. Depression of respiration and hypotension with loss of consciousness in late stages. Salicylate of **Physostigmine** is effective antidote.

Benzilonium Parasympatholytic with peripheral effects, toxic effects, etc. similar to **Atropine**. Used as antispasmodic for gastro-intestinal disorders and to reduce gastric acid secretion in peptic ulceration.

Benzocaine Weak local anaesthetic similar to **Lignocaine**. Used in proprietary preparations for sore throats.

Benzoctamine Anxiolytic. Actions, uses and adverse effects similar to **Diazepam**.

Benzoic acid Used topically for mild fungus infections of skin.

Benzoin Plant resin extract used as inhalation to reduce catarrh in upper respiratory tract and as topical skin preparation to reduce or prevent dryness and fissures.

Benzoylmetronidazole Antibacterial, formulated as suspension for those unable to swallow tablets. Otherwise identical to **Metronidazole**.

Benzoyl peroxide Antiseptic/keratolytic. Powder used in dusting powders and in creams and lotions in treatment of burns, skin ulcers, and acne.

Benzthiazide Diuretic, with actions similar to **Chlorothiazide**.

Benztropine Antispasmodic parasympatholytic used in parkinsonism. Similar to **Benzhexol**, but more potent and can be given by intramuscular injection. Particularly useful in treating drug-induced parkinsonism.

Benzydamine Analgesic with anti-inflammatory and antipyretic properties similar to **Acetylsalicylic acid**. Used topically as cream for musculoskeletal pains and as a mouthwash for sore throat. Overdosage by mouth has caused agitation, anxiety, hallucinations, and convulsions.

Benzyl benzoate Used as insect repellent, in treatment of scabies, and as antipruritic. May cause allergic rashes.

Benzyl nicotinate Vasodilator related to **Nicotinic acid**.

Benzylpenicillin Bactericidal antibiotic (see **Penicillins**). Unstable at acid pH, poorly active by mouth. Given parenterally. Active against most gram-positive and some gram-negative organisms. Inactivated by penicillinase. Adverse effects include hypersensitivity reactions, both immediate and delayed, and encephalopathy with convulsions if given intrathecally or in massive doses.

Bephenium Used in treatment of hookworms. Adverse effects include nausea, vomiting, and vertigo.

Betahistine Vasodilator with actions similar to **Histamine**. Used in Ménière's disease to reduce episodes of dizziness.

Betamethasone Potent synthetic **Corticosteroid** similar to **Dexamethasone**.

Betaxolol Beta-adrenoceptor blocking drug with cardioselectivity. Used as an antihypertensive. Adverse effects and precautions as for **Propranolol**.

Betazole Related to **Histamine**, with similar actions and uses.

Bethanechol Parasympathomimetic drug, with actions of **Acetylcholine**.

Bethanidine Adrenergic neurone blocking drug. Used in hypertension. Adverse effects as for **Guanethidine**.

Bezafibrate Reduces blood fats, with uses, interactions, and adverse effects similar to **Clofibrate**.

Bile salts Extracted from animal bile. Used to stimulate bile flow without increasing its bile salts and pigment contents (e.g., after biliary operations). Included in some compound preparations for treatment of biliary insufficiency, but of doubtful efficacy.

Biotin (Vitamin H) Found in liver, kidney, yeast, eggs, and milk. Until recently there was no known clinical deficiency state. Induced deficiency caused dermatitis, lassitude, anorexia, and parasthesiae. It is now known that several extremely rare inborn metabolic disorders present with similar symptoms and respond to biotin.

Bisacodyl Purgative that acts by stimulating sensory nerve endings in wall of large bowel. Available for oral and rectal use. Suppositories may cause mild burning sensation in the rectum.

Bismuth aluminate See **Bismuth antacids**.

Bismuth antacids Insoluble bismuth salts have weak antacid properties and are claimed to protect the stomach. Largely superseded by more effective antacids. Prolonged, excessive use may allow sufficient absorption to cause toxicity with kidney damage, liver damage, and CNS effects.

Bismuth carbonate See **Bismuth antacids**.

Bismuth formic iodide Topical anti-infective powder.

Bismuth oxide See **Bismuth antacids**.

Bismuth salicylate Bismuth salt administered by mouth for protective effect on stomach and bowels. Converted to **Bismuth** and **Sodium salicylate** in small intestine. Used as symptomatic treatment for indigestion, nausea, and diarrhoea.

Bismuth subgallate Insoluble powder used for eczema and as suppositories for haemorrhoids.

Bismuth subnitrate See **Bismuth antacids**.

Bleomycin Cytotoxic antibiotic used to treat lymphomas and solid tumours. Toxic effects include lung fibrosis and skin pigmentation.

Boric acid Weak anti-infective powder used in dusting powders, lotions, and ointments.

Bran Purgative, non-irritant. Byproduct of milling of wheat. Contains indigestible cellulose which increases intestinal bulk. Crude bran is unpalatable; processed bran is pleasant cereal. Large doses needed for effect. Danger of bowel obstruction if pre-existing bowel narrowing.

Bretylium Adrenergic neurone blocking drug with actions similar to **Guanethidine**. Used mainly in cardiac arrhythmias. Side effects have limited its use as antihypertensive.

Bromazepam Benzodiazepine anxiolytic, with actions and adverse effects similar to **Diazepam**.

Bromhexine Mucolytic, expectorant. Administered orally. Said to increase secretion of fluid by respiratory tract and to break down mucus. Used when viscid mucus is troublesome (e.g., chronic bronchitis). May cause gastro-intestinal side effects. Not to be given if there is pre-existing peptic ulceration.

Bromides CNS depressants, now largely superseded by safer drugs.

Bromocriptine Stimulates dopamine receptors. Used in treatment of acromegaly, for inhibition or suppression of lactation, and in conditions due to excessive prolactin secretion, including some cases of infertility. Adverse effects include nausea, hypotension, and cold extremities.

Brompheniramine Antihistamine, with actions similar to **Promethazine**.

Bronopol Antibacterial preservative used in topical preparations.

Buclizine Antihistamine/anti-emetic drug with actions similar to **Promethazine**.

Budesonide Synthetic **Corticosteroid** similar to **Dexamethasone**. Used by inhalation for treatment of asthma. Also applied intranasally for allergic rhinitis.

Bufexamac Topical, non-steroid anti-inflammatory/analgesic with actions similar to **Indomethacin**. Used in dermatitis and haemorrhoids.

Bufylline Bronchodilator, with actions similar to **Aminophylline**.

Bumetanide Potent diuretic, with actions and uses similar to **Frusemide**. Adverse effects similar to **Bendrofluazide**.

Bupivacaine Local anaesthetic similar to **Lignocaine**, but produces longer anaesthesia.

Buprenorphine Narcotic analgesic with antagonist properties for injection or as sublingual tablets. Actions, uses, and adverse effects similar to **Pentazocine**.

Busulphan Cytotoxic drug used in neoplastic disease, particularly myeloid leukaemia. Adverse effects include skin pigmentation, cataract, pulmonary fibrosis, and bone marrow depression.

Butacaine Local anaesthetic used by injection or by spray on to the mucosa of the nose and throat. Actions and adverse effects similar to **Lignocaine**.

Butethamate Sympathomimetic amine, with actions similar to **Ephedrine**.

Butobarbitone (c) Barbiturate hypnotic essentially like **Amylobarbitone**.

Butorphanol Analgesic injection, with actions and uses similar to **Morphine**, but has narcotic antagonist activity similar to **Naloxone**. May cause sedation, dizziness, nausea, changes in mood, and vivid dreams. Has low potential for dependence and addiction, and may precipitate withdrawal symptoms in narcotic addicts. May depress respiration and therefore caution is advised if used in patients with respiratory disease. **Naloxone**, but not **Nalorphine** or **Levallorphan**, may be used as antagonist.

Butoxyethyl nicotinate See **Nicotinic acid**.

Butriptyline Antidepressant, with actions and uses similar to **Imipramine**.

Butyl aminobenzoate Local anaesthetic for topical use.

C

Caffeine Active principle from tea and coffee, used as mild CNS stimulant. Adverse effects include restlessness, excitement, and dependence after prolonged excessive ingestion. Claimed to enhance the absorption and thus the effectiveness of **Ergotamine** in migraine. Its inclusion in many analgesic preparations is presumably to counteract any sedative effects and is of doubtful value.

Calamine Zinc carbonate used in dusting powders, creams, lotions, etc.

Calciferol See **Vitamin D**.

Calcitonin Hormone from thyroid glands, involved in control of calcium metabolism. Used in treatment of Paget's disease.

Calcitriol (1α,25-Dihydroxycholecalciferol) More potent active metabolite of **Vitamin D**.

Calcium carbonate Nonsystematic (nonabsorbable) antacid. Used in treatment of peptic ulceration where it produces longer neutralization of acid than **Sodium bicarbonate**. Frequent use may cause constipation. Small amounts are absorbed and in some subjects may cause renal stones (i.e. nephrocalcinosis).

Calcium gluconate Source of calcium for deficiency states.

Calcium iodide Used as expectorant.

Calcium lactate See **Calcium gluconate**.

Calcium polystyrene sulphonate Ion exchange resin used to treat electrolyte abnormalities by changing absorption or excretion in the gut.

Calcium sulphaloxate Sulphonamide antibacterial, with actions similar to **Sulphadimidine**. Very little absorbed. Used for prevention or treatment of mild infective diarrhoea.

Camphene See **Camphor**.

Camphor Used internally as carminative and externally as rubefacient.

Candicidin Antifungal antibiotic used locally for vaginal and skin infections.

Capreomycin Peptide antibiotic, mainly used in tuberculosis. Adverse effects include ototoxicity and nephrotoxicity.

Capsicum Essential oil used internally as carminative and externally as rubefacient.

Captopril Inhibits enzyme involved in formation of hormone concerned with maintenance of blood pressure. Used in treatment of hypertension resistant to other drugs. Adverse effects include hypotension, proteinuria, bone marrow depression, skin rashes, and loss of taste.

Caraway Essential oil used as carminative.

Carbachol Parasympathomimetic, with actions and adverse effects similar to **Acetylcholine**, but more prolonged. Used as miotic eye drops in glaucoma and for improvement of postoperative intestinal or bladder muscle tone.

Carbamazepine Anticonvulsant. Acts by suppressing epileptic discharges in the brain. Used in prevention of epilepsy and in suppression of pain in trigeminal neuralgia, but is not an analgesic. May cause drowsiness, blurred vision, dizziness, and gastro-intestinal upsets. Skin rashes and adverse effects on the liver and bone marrow are relatively common. Coma with convulsions in overdosage. No antidote; supportive treatment only.

Carbaryl Anticholinesterase. Used topically as an insecticide (e.g., for lice).

Carbenicillin **Penicillin** antibiotic, particularly active against gram-negative bacteria especially *Pseudomonas* and *Proteus*. Adverse effects as for **Benzylpenicillin**.

Carbenoxolone Used in treatment of gastric and duodenal ulcers and for mouth ulcers. Has **Aldosterone**-like actions. Adverse effects include oedema, hypertension, hypokalaemia, and muscle pain.

Carbidopa Similar actions to **Benserazide**.

Carbimazole Depresses formation of thyroid hormone. Used in treatment of hyperthyroidism. Adverse effects include allergic rashes, nausea, diarrhoea, blood abnormalities, and keratitis..

Carbinoxamine Antihistamine, with actions similar to **Promethazine**.

Carbocysteine Mucolytic used to reduce viscosity of sputum.

Carbromal Weak hypnotic. May produce dependence. Adverse effects include rashes and purpura. Chronic effects (bromism) include mental depression and slurring of speech. Acute intoxication produces respiratory failure.

Carfecillin Similar to **Carbenicillin**.

Carisoprodol Used to treat painful muscle spasm.

Carmellose Cellulose derivative employed in artificial tears and as a pharmaceutical aid in drug formulations.

Carmustine Intravenous cytotoxic, inactivates DNA, RNA, and several enzymes. Crosses the blood–brain barrier, thus useful for brain tumours as well as certain other neoplastic diseases. Rapidly degraded from the parent drug to active metabolites. Adverse effects include nausea, vomiting, burning sensation at injection site, renal and hepatic damage, and delayed bone marrow suppression.

Cascara Purgative from bark of buckthorn tree. Stimulates gut movement via the nerve plexus in the large bowel wall. Produces reddish-brown discoloration of urine and may cause excessive catharsis. Excreted in milk of lactating mothers and may cause diarrhoea in infants. Prolonged use causes black pigmentation in colon (melanosis coli).

Castor oil Purgative, with action upon small intestine as well as large intestine, useful when prompt evacuation is required (e.g., before bowel X-rays). Chronic use not recommended as it causes reduced absorption of nutrients. Also used topically on skin for its emollient effect.

Cefaclor Cephalosporin antibiotic. Orally active and has wider range of activity than earlier drugs of that group. Actions, uses, and adverse effects similar to **Cephalothin**.

Cefadroxil **Cephalosporin** antibiotic similar to **Cephalexin**.

Cefotaxime Broad-spectrum **Cephalosporin** antibiotic for injection, with actions, uses, and adverse effects similar to **Cephalothin**.

Cefoxitin Cephamycin antibiotic for injection. Related to the **Cephalosporins** with similar actions, uses, and adverse effects, but may have broader spectrum of activity.

Cefsoludin Injectable **Cephalosporin** antibiotic with narrow spectrum but specifically active against *Pseudomonas aeruginosa* infections. Dosage must be reduced in renal failure since this drug is excreted unchanged in the urine. Other adverse effects as for **Cephalothin**.

Ceftazidime **Cephalosporin** antibiotic for injection. Has wider range of antibacterial activity than earlier drugs of this group. Adverse effects similar to **Cephalothin**.

Ceftizoxime **Cephalosporin** antibiotic for injection. Has range of antibacterial activity similar to **Ceftazidime**. Adverse effects similar to **Cephalothin**.

Cefuroxime **Cephalosporin** antibiotic for injection. Has wider range of antibacterial activity than earlier drugs in this group. Actions, uses, and adverse effects similar to **Cephalothin**.

Centella asiatica Plant extract used in skin preparations to promote healing.

Cephalexin **Cephalosporin** antibiotic, with similar activity and adverse effects to **Cephalothin**, but well absorbed by mouth.

Cephaloridine **Cephalosporin** antibiotic, administered parenterally. May cause renal damage, particularly if given with **Frusemide**. Other adverse effects include hypersensitivity reactions.

Cephalosporins Bactericidal antibiotics that inhibit bacterial cell wall synthesis. Have similar basic structure to **Penicillins**, but are relatively resistant to penicillinase. Among this drug group, **Cephaloridine** alone has been clearly implicated as a cause of renal damage.

Cephalothin **Cephalosporin** antibiotic, particularly useful against penicillinase-producing *Staphylococcus aureus*. Must be given parenterally. Adverse effects mainly hypersensitivity reactions.

Cephamandole Newer **Cephalosporin** antibiotic for injection. Has wider range of antibacterial activity than earlier drugs of this group. Actions, uses, and adverse effects similar to **Cephalothin**.

Cephazolin **Cephalosporin** antibiotic similar to **Cephalexin**.

Cephradine **Cephalosporin** antibiotic similar to **Cephalexin**.

Ceratonia Powder prepared from the endosperm of the locust bean tree *(Ceratonia siliqua)*. Used as a mucilage to thicken feeds for children with diarrhoea.

Cetalkonium Topical disinfectant.

Cetomacrogol Emulsifying wax used in formulating oil-in-water emulsons.

Cetostearyl alcohol Mixture of solid alcohols used for emulsifying properties in oil-in-water formulations including preparations for protection of dry skin.

Cetrimide Topical disinfectant used in many skin preparations.

Cetyl alcohol Used in manufacture of ointments and creams.

Cetylpyridinium Topical disinfectant used in skin and mouth preparations.

Charcoal Used as adsorbant in first aid treatment of poisoning by drugs and toxins. Also used to treat diarrhoea.

Chenodeoxycholic acid Naturally occurring bile acid which prevents formation and aids dissolution of gall stones.

Chloral hydrate Hypnotic. Available only as a liquid. Converted by liver to trichloroethanol which causes generalized CNS depression. Used for insomnia, especially in children and the elderly. Relatively 'safe'. Addiction is rare. Interacts with oral anticoagulants increasing their effect and rate of elimination. Coma in overdosage. No antidote; treated by supportive measures.

Chlorambucil Cytotoxic drug related to **Mustine hydrochloride**. Used in neoplastic conditions of lymphoid tissues. Adverse effects include bone marrow depression.

Chloramphenicol Broad-spectrum bacteriostatic antibiotic, which should be reserved for treatment of typhoid fever and life-threatening infections. Adverse effects include aplastic anaemia. Produces 'grey baby syndrome' in neonates and premature babies.

Chlorbutol Antibacterial and antifungal preservative for topical applications.

Chlorcyclizine Antihistamine, with similar actions and adverse effects to **Promethazine**. Used mainly as an anti-emetic.

Chlordantoin Topical antifungal agent.

Chlordiazepoxide Benzodiazepine anxiolytic similar to **Diazepam** but less hypnotic and less anticonvulsant activity. Used in treatment of anxiety.

Chlorexolone Diuretic, with actions, uses, and adverse effects similar to **Bendrofluazide**.

Chlorhexidine Topical disinfectant used in skin preparations, urethral catheterization, cytoscopy, and as preservative in eye drops.

Chlormethiazole Sedative/hypnotic/anticonvulsant. Depressant action on CNS. Used for sedation or hypnosis in agitated or confused patients especially the elderly. Also for treatment of acute withdrawal symptoms in alcoholics and drug addicts and control of sustained epileptic fits (status epilepticus). May cause tingling in nose and sneezing. Effects potentiated by **Chlorpromazine, Haloperidol** and related drugs. Coma with respiratory depression in overdosage. No antidote. Symptomatic treatment is adequate.

Chlormezanone Anxiolytic, muscle relaxant. Sometimes used as a hypnotic. Actions similar to **Meprobamate**. Adverse effects include drowsiness, dizziness, headache, skin rashes and jaundice.

Chlorocresol Disinfectant used in sterilizing solutions and as a preservative in creams.

Chlorofluoromethane Aerosol propellant for drugs administered by inhalation. Also used as a spray for muscle pain where it produces local anaesthesia due to intense coldness.

Chlorophenoxyethanol Topical antibacterial.

Chloroquine Antimalarial agent, which has also been used in rheumatoid arthritis. Adverse effects include skin pigmentation, alopecia, neuropathy, and corneal and retinal damage.

Chlorothiazide Thiazide diuretic similar to **Bendrofluazide**.

Chlorothymol Topical antiseptic.

Chlorotrianisene Synthetic female sex hormone used in menopausal symptoms and to suppress lactation. Adverse effects similar to **Oestradiol**.

Chloroxylenol Topical disinfectant used chiefly on skin.

Chlorphenesin Topical antibacterial/antifungal agent.

Chlorpheniramine Antihistamine, with actions, uses, and adverse effects similar to **Promethazine**.

Chlorphenoxamine Antihistamine similar to **Promethazine** used in Parkinson's disease.

Chlorphentermine (c) Anorectic, sympathomimetic amine. Actions and adverse effects similar to **Diethylpropion**.

Chlorpromazine Phenothiazine tranquillizer. Causes selective depression of the brain structures responsible for control of behaviour and wakefulness. Has anticholinergic alpha-adrenergic blocking and dopaminergic effects amongst other pharmacological effects. Used in psychotic disorders, particularly schizophrenia and agitated depression; in terminal illness to enhance analgesia; to control nausea and vomiting; and for hiccups. Adverse effects include postural hypotension, dry mouth, blurred vision, involuntary movements, cholestatic jaundice, photosensitivity, and deposits in lens and cornea. Used only with caution in liver disease and epilepsy (may precipitate convulsions). In overdosage causes coma, involuntary movements, convulsions, hypotension, and arrhythmias. No antidote; supportive treatment only.

Chlorpropamide Oral antidiabetic drug that stimulates pancreatic insulin release in maturity-onset diabetes mellitus. Adverse effects include hypoglycaemia, allergic reactions, jaundice, and flushing with alcohol. Action may be potentiated by salicylates and sulphonamides. Sometimes used in diabetes insipidus.

Chlorprothixene Phenothiazine tranquillizer essentially similar to **Chlorpromazine**.

Chlorquinaldol Topical antibacterial/antifungal similar to **Hydroxyquinoline**. Used in skin infections.

Chlortetracycline Bacteriostatic antibiotic, with actions, adverse effects, and interactions similar to **Tetracycline**.

Chlorthalidone Diuretic essentially similar to **Bendrofluazide**.

Cholesterol Natural fatty constituent of all animal cells and a precursor of steroids. Used topically in creams for soothing and water-absorbing properties.

Cholestyramine Resin that binds bile salts in gut. Used in pruritus associated with jaundice and to reduce blood cholesterol. Adverse effects include nausea, diarrhoea, and constipation.

Choline magnesium trisalicylate A mixture of **Choline salicylate** and magnesium salicylate with actions, uses, and adverse effects similar to **Acetysalicylic acid**.

Choline salicylate Similar actions to **Acetylsalicylic acid**.

Choline theophyllinate Oral preparation of **Theophylline**, with actions similar to **Aminophylline**. Main use is in chronic bronchitis.

Chorionic gonadotrophin Hormone produced in the placenta. Used in treatment of anovulatory infertility and failure of development of the testes or ovaries. May cause fluid retention and therefore used with caution if there is evidence of cardiac or renal failure.

Chymotrypsin Animal pancreatic enzyme used to reduce soft tissue inflammation, particularly associated with trauma. Adverse effects include allergic reactions.

Ciclacillin **Penicillin** antibiotic with broad spectrum similar to **Ampicillin**, but improved absorption from gastro-intestinal tract. Uses and adverse effects similar to **Ampicillin**.

Cimetidine Selectively blocks histamine receptors mediating gastric acid secretion. Used in peptic ulceration and gastric hyperacidity, oesophageal reflux and prophylaxis of gastro-intestinal bleeding in seriously ill patients. Adverse effects include diarrhoea, dizziness, rash and breast enlargement in males. Danger of CNS depression and confusional states in renal failure, the elderly, or seriously ill patients.

Cinchocaine Local anaesthetic with actions similar to **Lignocaine**.

Cinnarizine Antihistamine similar to **Promethazine**, chiefly used in treatment of vertigo and vomiting.

Cinoxacin Antibacterial for urinary infections. Actions and adverse effects similar to **Nalidixic acid**.

Cisplatin Cytotoxic platinum compound used in treatment of metastatic testicular and ovarian tumours. May cause renal damage, ototoxicity, bone marrow suppression, nausea, vomiting, and allergic reactions.

Clavulanic acid Inhibits the enzyme penicillinase which inactivates penicillin antibiotics. Used with **Amoxycillin** to increase its spectrum of activity.

Clemastine Antihistamine, with actions and uses similar to **Promethazine**, but with less sedative effects.

Clemizole Antihistamine similar to **Promethazine**.

Clidinium Actions similar to **Atropine**. Used in treatment of peptic ulcer and gastric hyperacidity.

Clindamycin Antibiotic, with actions and adverse effects similar to **Lincomycin**, but better absorbed.

Clioquinol Used in treatment of gut amoebiasis and to protect against gut infections, used topically for skin infections. Prolonged large oral doses may produce neuropathy.

Clobazam Benzodiazepine anxiolytic with actions, uses, and adverse effects similar to **Diazepam**. May also be used for long-term anticonvulsant therapy, similar to **Clonazepam**.

Clobetasol Topical **Corticosteroid** for psoriasis and eczema.

Clobetasone Topical **Corticosteroid** for psoriasis and eczema.

Clofazimine Antileprotic/anti-inflammatory, used for control of reactions occurring with **Dapsone** treatment. Adverse effects include skin pigmentation, red urine, and diarrhoea.

Clofibrate Reduces blood cholesterol and fats. Used in patients with raised levels of these constituents. Adverse effects include nausea, diarrhoea, muscle pain, and weakness. Potentiates anticoagulants.

Clomiphene Sex hormone used in infertility due to failure of ovulation. Acts both on the pituitary gonadotrophic hormones and on the ovary permitting ovulation. Should not be used in liver failure or if patient has ovarian cysts. Danger of multiple births, especially at higher doses.

Clomipramine Antidepressant drug, with actions and uses similar to **Imipramine**.

Clomocycline Bacteriostatic antibiotic, with actions, adverse effects, and interactions similar to **Tetracycline**.

Clonazepam Benzodiazepine anticonvulsant similar to **Diazepam** but has greater anticonvulsant activity. Used intravenously for control of status epilepticus, orally for prevention of all types of epilepsy.

Clonidine Reduces sympathetic activity by central action, and reduces vascular reactivity. Used in hypertension and in migraine. Antihypertensive effect blocked by tricyclic antidepressants. Adverse effects include sedation, depression, dryness of mouth, fluid retention. Rapid withdrawal may be associated with 'rebound hypertension'.

Clopamide Diuretic essentially similar to **Bendrofluazide**.

Clopenthixol Major tranquillizer with actions similar to **Chlorpromazine**. Used in treatment of schizophrenia. Sedation and hypotension are predictable adverse effects. Extrapyramidal (parkinsonian) symptoms are less frequent than with **Chlorpromazine**.

Clorazepate Anxiolytic, with actions, uses, and adverse effects similar to **Diazepam**. Long-acting and has sedative effects, so is best given at night. Metabolized to desmethyldiazepam, an active metabolite of **Diazepam**.

Clorexolone Diuretic essentially similar to **Bendrofluazide**.

Clorprenaline Bronchodilator similar to **Ephedrine**.

Clotrimazole Antifungal agent used topically for skin infections with *Candida*.

Cloxacillin Penicillinase-resistant **Penicillin** with actions and adverse effects similar to **Benzylpenicillin**. Use restricted to treatment of penicillinase-producing *Staphylococcus aureus* infections.

Coal tar Keratolytic used in topical preparations for eczema and psoriasis.

Cobalt tetracemate (Cobalt edetate) Antidote for cyanide poisoning. Binds with cyanide and prevents its effects upon cell metabolism.

Cocaine (c) Local anaesthetic. Stabilizes nerve cell membranes to prevent impulse transmission. Little used except topically in eye or respiratory passages. Frequent use may cause corneal ulceration. Stimulates CNS with euphoria and consequent risk of addiction. Chronic misuse leads to delusions, hallucinations, and paranoia.

Co-codamol Contains **Codeine** and **Paracetamol** in a fixed ratio.

Co-codaprin Contains **Codeine** and **Acetylsalicylic acid** in a fixed ratio.

Co-danthramer Contains **Danthron** and **Poloxamer '188'** in a fixed ratio.

Co-danthrusate Contains **Danthron** and **Dioctyl sodium sulphosuccinate** in a fixed ratio.

Codeine Weak narcotic analgesic. Used for somatic (deep) pain often combined with **Acetylsalicylic acid** or **Paracetamol**. Also causes constipation and suppresses the cough reflex. May therefore be used as an anti-diarrhoeal and in cough mixtures. Addiction very unusual. Coma with respiratory depression in overdosage. **Naloxone** is antidote.

Co-dergocrine See **Dihydroergotoxine**.

Co-dydramol Contains **Dihydrocodeine** and **Paracetamol** in a fixed ratio.

Colaspase See **L-Asparaginase**.

Colchicine Used for relief of pain in acute gout. Adverse effects include nausea, vomiting, colicky pain, and diarrhoea.

Colestipol Ion exchange resin which lowers plasma cholesterol levels through binding with bile acids in the intestinal lumen. Used as an adjunct to diet in treatment of high cholesterol levels. May cause constipation. Must be taken mixed with water or may cause oesophageal damage.

Colistin Antibiotic: see **Polymyxin B**.

Colophony Resin used in protective topical preparations.

Compound gentian infusion Bitter extract from the dried root of *Gentiana lutea*. Used to stimulate gastric acid secretion and thus to stimulate appetite.

Copper acetate Used topically for its astringent properties.

Copper sulphate Used as an emetic, together with iron in treatment of anaemia, and as astringent in topical preparations. Large doses may cause copper poisoning. Syrup of **Ipecacuanha** is generally considered a safer emetic.

Co-proxamol Contains **Dextropropoxyphene** and **Paracetamol** in a fixed ratio.

Corticosteroids General term to include natural and synthetic steroids, with actions similar to **Hydrocortisone**, which is produced in the adrenal cortex. They possess anti-inflammatory and salt-retaining properties. Adverse effects include oedema, hypertension, diabetes, bone thinning with fractures, muscle wasting, infections, and psychosis.

Corticotrophin Pituitary hormone that controls functions of adrenal cortex.

Cortisone Naturally occurring adrenal (glucocorticoid) steroid hormone. Has effects upon fat, protein and carbohydrate metabolism, and possesses marked anti-inflammatory activity. Used for replacement therapy in adrenal insufficiency, anti-inflammatory activity in a wide range of conditions, and immunosuppression after organ transplantation or in certain leukaemias. Adverse effects include retention of salt and water, fulminating infections, osteoporosis, peptic ulceration, muscle wasting, hypertension, diabetes mellitus, weight gain, moon face, cataracts, and psychiatric disturbance. On withdrawal of large doses after long periods of treatment there may be failure of the natural adrenal hormone secretion.

Co-trimazine Antibacterial. Combination of **Sulphadiazine** and **Trimethoprim**. Actions and adverse effects similar to **Co-trimoxazole** but **Sulphadiazine** is metabolized less than **Sulphamethoxazole** resulting in higher drug concentrations in kidneys and urine. Used for urinary tract infections.

Co-trimoxazole Antimicrobial. Combination of **Sulphamethoxazole** and **Trimethoprim**. Broad antibacterial spectrum, active against typhoid fever. Adverse effects include rashes and blood dyscrasias.

Cresol Antiseptic. Used as disinfectant or preservative and also as an inhalant for relief of congestion in bronchitis, asthma, and the common cold. If ingested in concentrated solutions, there may be local corrosion, depression of the CNS, and damage to the liver and kidneys.

Crotamiton Topical treatment for scabies.

Cyanocobalamin Largely replaced by **Hydroxocobalamin**.

Cyclandelate Peripheral vasodilator acting by relaxation of muscle in blood vessel walls. Used in treatment of peripheral vascular insufficiency (e.g., Raynaud's syndrome). Also used in cases of impaired mental function due to cerebrovascular disease. May cause dizziness, flushing, headache, and nausea.

Cyclizine Antihistamine, with actions similar to **Promethazine**. Main use as anti-emetic.

Cyclobarbitone (c) Barbiturate hypnotic, with actions, uses, and adverse effects similar to **Amylobarbitone**.

Cyclofenil Sex hormone used in treatment of infertility due to failure of ovulation. Contraindications and adverse effects similar to **Clomiphene**.

Cyclopenthiazide Thiazide diuretic similar to **Bendrofluazide**.

Cyclopentolate Anticholinergic, with actions and adverse effects similar to **Atropine** but with more rapid onset and shorter duration. Used as eye drops to dilate the pupil and to assist optical refraction.

Cyclophosphamide Cytotoxic used in wide variety of neoplastic diseases. Activated by metabolism in the liver and excreted mainly in the urine. Adverse effects include baldness, cystitis, and renal and bone marrow toxicity.

Cyclopropane Potent inhalational anaesthetic. Used to induce anaesthesia in paediatric and obstetric practice.

Cycloserine Antibiotic used in tuberculosis and in *Escherichia coli* and *Proteus* infections. Adverse effects include ataxia, drowsiness, and convulsions.

Cyclosporin Potent immunosuppressant antibiotic used to prevent rejection after organ and tissue transplantation. Adverse effects include impairment of liver and renal function.

Cycrimine Parasympatholytic used in treatment of parkinsonism. Similar actions, etc. to **Benzhexol**.

Cyproheptadine Antihistamine similar to **Promethazine**. Stimulates appetite.

Cyproterone Hormone with antiandrogenic and some progestogenic activity used in the treatment of prostatic carcinoma. Has also been used in sexual disorders in the male, acne, and hirsutism. May cause gynaecomastia, galactorrhoea, sedation, mood changes, altered hair pattern, skin rashes, weight gain, headache, anaemia, and fluctuations in blood pressure. Also avoided in liver disease, thromboembolic disorders, diabetes, and immature youths..

Cysteamine Antidote for severe poisoning due to **Paracetamol** where it is thought to prevent liver damage by reducing the concentration of a toxic metabolite. Must be given by intravenous injection and may cause marked adverse effects including protracted nausea and vomiting. Should not be given more than ten hours after the overdose as it may exacerbate liver damage.

Cytarabine (Cytosine arabinoside) Antiviral agent used systemically for herpes encephalitis. Cytotoxic, used in treatment of leukaemia and Hodgkin's disease. Adverse effects include bone marrow depression.

Cytosine arabinoside See **Cytarabine**.

D

Dacarbazine Cytotoxic. May cause bone marrow suppression.

Dactinomycin See **Actinomycin D**.

Dakin's solution Contains calcium hypochlorite, **Sodium bicarbonate**, **Boric acid**. Used as wound disinfectant.

Danazol Used in endocrine disturbances where pituitary control of gonad hormone production is required.

Danthron Purgative, with actions, etc. similar to **Cascara**.

Dantrolene Used in control of skeletal muscle spasticity. Adverse effects include sedation, weakness, and diarrhoea.

Dapsone Sulphone drug used in treatment of leprosy. Adverse effects include allergic dermatitis, nausea, vomiting, tachycardia, haemolytic anaemia, and liver damage.

Daunomycin See **Daunorubicin**.

Daunorubicin (Rubidomycin, Daunomycin) Cytotoxic antibiotic used in neoplastic disease. Adverse effects include cardiotoxicity and bone marrow depression.

Debrisoquine Adrenergic neurone blocking drug used in hypertension. Adverse effects as for **Guanethidine**.

Deglycyrrhizinised liquorice Mild anti-inflammatory agent. Used in treatment of peptic ulcer. Adverse effects include oedema and hypertension.

Dehydrocholic acid Used to stimulate secretion of bile flow without increasing its content of bile solids (e.g., after surgery of biliary tract).

Demecarium Anticholinesterase used by instillation into eye in glaucoma. Actions those of **Acetylcholine**.

Demeclocycline See **Demethylchlortetracycline**.

Demethylchlortetracycline Bacteriostatic antibiotic with actions, adverse effects, and interactions similar to **Tetracycline**.

Deoxycortone Potent salt-retaining **Corticosteroid** used by injection, implant, or sublingually in adrenal insufficiency. Adverse effects as for **Corticosteroids**.

Deptropine Antihistamine similar to **Promethazine**.

Dequalinium Topical antibacterial/antifungal used in oral infections.

Deserpidine See **Reserpine**.

Desferrioxamine Binds with iron. Used orally and parenterally in treatment of acute iron poisoning and in conditions associated with excessive iron storage in tissues, where it increases urinary iron excretion. Adverse effects include allergic reactions.

Desipramine Antidepressant. Active metabolite of **Imipramine**, whose actions and adverse effects it shares.

Desmopressin Synthetic form of **Vasopressin** for use nasally in diabetes insipidus.

Desogestrel Sex hormone, with actions and adverse effects similar to **Progesterone**. Used for oral contraception in combination with an oestrogenic hormone.

Desonide Topical corticosteroid for psoriasis and eczema.

Desoxymethasone **Corticosteroid** for topical skin use. Actions and adverse effects similar to **Dexamethasone**.

Deoxyribonuclease Animal pancreatic enzyme used to resolve clots and exudates associated with trauma and inflammation.

Dexamethasone Potent synthetic **Corticosteroid** with actions, etc. similar to **Cortisone**. Anti-inflammatory activity is much increased in potency, with no increase in salt and water-retaining activity.

Dexamphetamine (c) See **Amphetamine**.

Dexbrompheniramine Antihistamine with actions, uses, and adverse effects similar to **Brompheniramine**.

Dextranomer Spherical beads of dextran for surface application to skin wounds. Takes up fluid exudate by capillary action and aids removal of bacteria and tissue debris, thus improving wound healing.

Dextrans Polysaccharides used intravenously instead of blood or plasma to maintain blood volume and assist capillary flow. Used also as a lubricant in drops for dry eyes. Adverse effects include allergic reactions.

Dextromethorphan Cough suppressant. Adverse effects include slight psychic dependence and abuse.

Dextromoramide (c) Narcotic analgesic essentially similar to **Morphine** but more reliable when taken by mouth. Useful in the management of severe chronic pain in terminal disease.

Dextropropoxyphene Weak narcotic analgesic with potency less than **Codeine**. Used in moderate pain, commonly with **Paracetamol** when the latter drug is not fully effective. In normal doses, causes less nausea, vomiting, and constipation than codeine. Coma with depressed respiration in overdosage. **Naloxone** is antagonist.

Dextrose Carbohydrate used orally or intravenously as a source of calories in cases of undernutrition. Readily absorbed from the gastro-intestinal tract. Metabolized by energy-producing pathways or stored in the liver as glycogen. Concentrated solutions by mouth may cause nausea and vomiting, intravenously may cause thrombophlebitis.

Dextrothyroxine Lipid-lowering drug. Reduces plasma cholesterol concentrations, but may cause tachycardia and angina in patients with ischaemic heart disease. Contraindicated in severe liver or kidney disease.

Diamorphine (Heroin) (c) Narcotic analgesic similar to **Morphine**. Less likely to cause nausea, vomiting, constipation, and hypotension, but greater euphorant action makes it more addicting and liable to greater abuse.

Diamthazole Topical antifungal agent. Adverse effects include convulsions if absorbed.

Diazepam Benzodiazepine minor tranquillizer (anxiolytic)/hypnotic with anticonvulsant properties. Acts centrally on the limbic system. Used in treatment of anxiety and as a hypnotic. Useful also in reduction of muscle tone in spasticity and as an anticonvulsant given intravenously for status epilepticus. May cause ataxia, nystagmus and sedation. May impair psychomotor performance. Caution required if driving or operating machinery. Coma in overdosage but little respiratory depression. No antidote. Supportive treatment is adequate.

Diazoxide Used to reduce blood pressure in severe hypertension and to increase blood sugar level in hypoglycaemia. Adverse effects include excessive hair growth, nausea, vomiting, oedema, diabetes, and hypotension.

Dibromopropamidine Topical antibacterial/antifungal.

Dichloralphenazone Hypnotic. Combination of **Chloral hydrate** and **Phenazone**. Available as tablets and elixir. Converted back to parent compounds by the liver. Used for insomnia especially in children and the elderly. Relatively 'safe'. Addiction is rare, but rashes and blood disorders may be caused by **Phenazone**.

Dichlorofluoromethane See **Chlorofluoromethane**.

Dichlorophen Used in treatment of tapeworms. Adverse effects include nausea, vomiting, and bowel colic.

Dichlorphenamide Used in treatment of respiratory failure from chronic bronchitis and in glaucoma. Adverse effects include electrolyte imbalance.

Diclofenac Non-steroid anti-inflammatory/analgesic/antipyretic used in treatment of rheumatoid arthritis and osteoarthritis. Adverse effects include gastro-intestinal upsets, headache, and dizziness.

Dicophane Insecticide used as dusting powder and lotion for fleas and lice. Very toxic if absorbed.

Dicoumarol Anticoagulant, with actions, interactions, and adverse effects similar to **Warfarin**.

Dicyclomine Parasympatholytic used in spasm of gastro-intestinal and urinary tracts and to reduce gastric acid in peptic ulceration. Actions, etc. similar to **Atropine** but weaker.

Dienoestrol Synthetic female sex hormone used for menopausal symptoms and for suppressing lactation. Adverse effects include nausea, vaginal bleeding, and oedema.

Diethylamine salicylate Rubefacient with actions similar to **Salicylic acid**.

Diethylcarbamazine Used in filariasis. Adverse effects include anorexia, nausea, vomiting. Allergic reactions may accompany release of foreign proteins on death of the worms.

Diethylpropion (c) Anorectic/sympathomimetic amine. Actions those of **Amphetamine** but less central stimulation and abuse potential.

Diflucortolone **Corticosteroid** for topical use in inflammatory skin conditions. Actions and adverse effects similar to **Cortisone**.

Diflunisal Analgesic related to **Acetylsalicylic acid**, but with longer duration of action and no effects on blood platelet function. May cause gastro-intestinal symptoms including ulceration and bleeding, although less common than with **Acetylsalicylic acid**. Should not be used if there is a history of hypersensitivity to **Acetylsalicylic acid**.

Digitalis Crude foxglove extract, with same actions, etc. as **Digoxin** but content of active drug is less reliable.

Digitoxin Foxglove derivative, with similar actions, etc. to **Digoxin**.

Digoxin Foxglove derivative. Increases force of contraction of heart and slows heart rate, thus making cardiac function more efficient. Used in heart failure and certain abnormal heart rhythms. Influenced by serum potassium levels and by kidney function. In therapeutic overdose, causes vomiting, abdominal pain, diarrhoea, impaired colour vision, slow heart rate, and abnormal heart rhythms.

Dihydrocodeine Mild narcotic analgesic similar to **Codeine**, but more potent in relief of pain and more likely to cause constipation. (c) if given by injection.

Dihydroergocornine See **Dihydroergotoxine**.

Dihydroergocristine See **Dihydroergotoxine**.

Dihydroergokryptine See **Dihydroergotoxine**.

Dihydroergotamine For migraine. Drops, tablets, or intramuscular injection. Used both for prevention and for symptomatic treatment. Has vasoconstrictor effects similar to **Ergotamine** but milder and with much reduced tendency to hypertension or effects on the uterus. No evidence of ergotism on prolonged or excessive use.

Dihydroergotoxine Mixture of **Dihydroergocornine, Dihydroergocristine,** and **Dihydroergokryptine**–ergot derivatives that are alpha-adrenoceptor blockers and vasodilators–used in peripheral and cerebral vascular disease. Adverse effects include nausea and nasal stuffiness.

Dihydrostreptomycin Antibiotic, with actions similar to **Streptomycin**, but more toxic to hearing.

Dihydrotachysterol Closely related to **Vitamin D** and has similar actions. Used in treatment of rickets and osteomalacia resistant to vitamin D. Also used in treatment of osteodystrophy due to chronic renal failure and in hypoparathyroidism. Contraindicated in hypercalcaemia, where it may cause ectopic calcification and renal failure.

Di-iodohydroxyquinoline Used orally for amoebiasis and topically as skin antiseptic.

Diloxanide Used in the treatment of intestinal amoebiasis, usually in combination with other drugs. Adverse effects include flatulence, vomiting, pruritus.

Diltiazem Antianginal drug that acts by blocking influx of calcium ions into cardiac muscle. Adverse effects include bradycardia, headache, and ankle swelling.

Dimenhydrinate Antihistamine/anti-emetic with actions similar to **Promethazine**.

Dimercaprol Binds to heavy metal. Used parenterally in treatment of heavy metal poisoning to increase urinary metal excretion. Adverse effects include nausea, vomiting, and hypertension.

Dimethicone Silicone used in protective creams and in antacid preparations.

Dimethindene Antihistamine similar to **Promethazine**.

Dimethisoquin Topical local anaesthetic used in lotions and ointments. Adverse effects include allergy and eye irritation.

Dimethyl sulphoxide Used as a solvent in pharmaceutical manufacture. Used alone to reduce inflammation, for example, in the bladder.

Dinoprost (Prostaglandin $F_2\alpha$) Used for induction of abortion.

Dinoprostone (Prostaglandin E_2) Used for induction of abortion.

Dioctyl sodium sulphosuccinate Purgative. Lowers surface tension of faecal mass allowing water to penetrate and soften faecal matter. Should not be given together with mineral oil laxatives (e.g., **Liquid paraffin**) as this drug may enhance absorption of the oil.

Diphenhydramine Antihistamine drug, with actions similar to **Promethazine**.

Diphenoxylate Reduces gut motility. Used in control of diarrhoea. Related to **Morphine**; adverse effects include drowsiness, euphoria, respiratory depression, coma, and dependence.

Diphenylpyraline Antihistamine similar to **Promethazine**.

Dipipanone (c) Narcotic analgesic essentially similar to **Methadone**.

Dipivefvrin Pro-drug, metabolized to **Adrenaline** after absorption. Used as eye drops for chronic open-angle glaucoma where the pro-drug passes through the cornea more readily than adrenaline. May cause transitory stinging of the eyes.

Diprophylline Bronchodilator, with actions similar to **Aminophylline**.

Dipyridamole Used in treatment of angina. Reduces platelet stickiness. Adverse effects include flushing, headache, and hypotension.

Disopyramide Used in abnormal heart rhythms. Adverse effects include dry mouth, blurred vision, and urinary hesitancy.

Distigmine Anticholinesterase: see **Neostigmine**.

Disulfiram Blocks alcohol metabolism at stage of acetaldehyde. Produces nausea, vomiting, severe headache, chest pain, dyspnoea, hypotension, and collapse if taken before alcohol. Used in treatment of alcoholism. Other adverse effects include impotence, neuropathy, and interference with anticoagulant activity of **Warfarin**.

Dithranol Used topically in psoriasis and other chronic skin conditions where it is thought to act by reducing the rate of skin cell formation. Adverse effects include staining of clothes and severe irritation to the eyes and skin.

Dobutamine Synthetic beta-adrenoceptor agonist chemically similar to **Isoprenaline**. Stimulates cardiac beta-adrenoceptors directly causing an increase in cardiac output with less increase in cardiac rate than with **Isoprenaline**. Used as infusion in treatment of shock. Unlike **Dopamine** does not cause constriction of peripheral blood vessels and rise in blood pressure but lacks the favourable effect of the latter on renal blood flow. May cause cardiac arrhythmias, but less frequent than with **Isoprenaline**.

Docusate sodium Laxative. Promotes water penetration into faeces with softening and increased rate of transit along large bowel.

Domiphen Topical disinfectant used in skin and mouth preparations.

Domperidone Anti-emetic, with dopamine antagonist actions similar to **Metoclopramide**. Used to control nausea and vomiting due to cancer chemotherapy. Adverse effects include drowsiness, involuntary movements, and cardiac dysrhythmias.

Dopamine Naturally occurring precursor of **Noradrenaline** that possesses sympathomimetic properties in its own right. Used intravenously in treatment of shock where it increases cardiac output with less risk of arrhythmias than **Isoprenaline**. Unlike **Dobutamine** or **Isoprenaline** has a vasodilator action on blood vessels to kidneys and may help to improve kidney function. Larger doses may cause peripheral vasoconstriction with a rise in pressure (see **Dobutamine**).

Dothiepin Tricyclic antidepressant, with actions, uses, etc. similar to **Imipramine**. Also has mild tranquillizing action, which may be useful in agitated depression. May cause extrapyramidal adverse effects.

Doxapram CNS stimulant used to stimulate respiration. Adverse effects include convulsions and abnormal heart rhythms.

Doxepin Tricyclic antidepressant, with actions, uses, etc. similar to **Impiramine**. Also has mild tranquillizing effect which may relieve anxiety associated with depression.

Doxorubicin Cytotoxic antibiotic used in neoplastic disease. Adverse effects include bone marrow depression, cardiotoxicity, and gastro-intestinal disturbances.

D-Xylose Sugar similar to glucose. Readily absorbed from the normal small intestine but has low rate of metabolism with consequent excretion of approximately 30 percent unchanged in the urine. Used as a test for intestinal malabsorption since lower absorption results in lower levels in the urine. May cause diarrhoea, nausea, and abdominal discomfort.

Doxycycline Bacteriostatic antibiotic, with actions, adverse effects, and interactions similar to **Tetacycline**. Unlike other tetracyclines, is not excreted by kidneys. Therefore used where renal impairment is a complication. The capsule formulation is apt to stick to the oesophageal mucosa where it dissolves and causes mucosal damage due to high acidity. A soluble formulation is available.

Doxylamine Antihistamine similar to **Promethazine**.

Droperidol Butyrophenone tranquillizer, with actions and adverse effects similar to **Haloperidol**. Used in combination with analgesics such as **Phenoperidine** to maintain the patient in a state of neuroleptanalgesia–calm and indifferent while conscious and able to cooperate with the surgeon.

Drostanolone Anabolic steroid given by intramuscular injection. Adverse effects as for **Testosterone**.

Dydrogesterone Actions similar to **Progesterone**, but does not inhibit ovulation and does not have contraceptive effect.

Dyflos Organophosphorus, long-acting anticholinesterase, with actions, etc. similar to **Physostigmine**.

E

Econazole Antifungal agent, with actions, uses, and adverse effects similar to **Miconazole**.

Ecothiopate Anticholinesterase similar to **Dyflos**.

Edrophonium Short-acting anticholinesterase, with actions similar to **Physostigmine**. Used in diagnosis of myasthenia gravis.

Embramine Antihistamine similar to **Promethazine**.

Emepronium Parasympatholytic, with actions, toxic effects similar to **Atropine**. Used to reduce tone in the urinary bladder when this is responsible for pain and frequency. May cause oesophageal ulceration if swallowed with insufficient fluid.

Emetine Anti-amoebic agent given by subcutaneous injection. Adverse effects include nausea, vomiting, hypotension, and cardiac arrhythmias.

Enalapril Antihypertensive, with actions, uses, and adverse effects similar to **Captopril**.

Enflurane Inhalation anaesthetic similar to **Halothane**.

Ephedrine Sympathomimetic amine with alpha and beta-adrenoceptor effects. Bronchodilator used in bronchial asthma. Also as mydriatic and nasal decongestant. Adverse effects include tachycardia, anxiety, and insomnia.

Epirubicin Cytotoxic antibiotic with uses, actions, and adverse effects similar to **Doxorubicin**.

Epoprostenol (Prostacyclin, PGI_2) Endogenously produced prostaglandin with potent vasodilator properties. Administered intravenously. Inhibits platelet aggregation. Preserves platelet function during cardiac bypass procedures and charcoal haemoperfusion. May be used as anticoagulant, alternative to heparin in renal dialysis. Adverse effects include headache, flushing, hypotension.

Epsilon-aminocaproic acid Antifibrinolytic agent used to reverse effects of **Streptokinase** or other fibrinolytic activity.

Epsom salts See **Magnesium sulphate**.

Ergometrine Derivative of ergot–a fungus which grows on rye. Causes contraction of uterine muscle. Used in obstetrics after delivery of the baby to prevent or reduce maternal haemorrhage. Adverse effects as for **Ergotamine**.

Ergotamine Ergot derivative similar to **Ergometrine** but with vasoconstricting and alpha-adrenoceptor blocking activity. Used in treatment of migraine by oral, intramuscular, sublingual, aerosol, or suppository routes. Adverse effects incluse nausea, vomiting, headache, convulsions, and cold extremities.

Erythromycin Bactericidal antibiotic, with spectrum of activity similar to **Benzylpenicillin**, plus some strains of *Haemophilus influenzae* and mycoplasmas. Adverse effects include diarrhoea and liver damage with jaundice.

Eserine See **Physostigmine**.

Essential oils Volatile oils taken orally for carminative effects in gastric discomfort. Induce a feeling of warmth with increased salivation. Large doses are irritant and may cause both gastro-intestinal symptoms and inflammation of the urinary tract.

Estramustine phosphate Cytotoxic drug used in neoplastic disease. Adverse effects include lower abdominal burning sensation and bone marrow depression.

Etafedrine Similar to **Ephedrine**.

Etamiphyllin Bronchodilator, with actions similar to **Aminophylline**.

Ethacrynic acid Potent diuretic. Action and uses similar to **Frusemide**. Adverse effects similar to **Bendrofluazide**. May also cause transient deafness.

Ethambutol Anti-tuberculous drug. Well tolerated but high doses toxic to optic nerve, producing central or periaxial retrobulbar neuritis.

Ethamivan Respiratory stimulant essentially similar to **Nikethamide**. May be used in respiratory depression of the newborn.

Ethamsylate Haemostatic agent used to control surgical and menstrual blood loss.

Ethanolamine Sclerosing agent used in the injection treatment of varicose veins. Contraindicated if there is thrombophlebitis. May cause hypersensitivity allergic reactions.

Ethchlorvynol Tertiary alcohol. Sedative/hypnotic. Rapid but short-lived general depressant action on CNS. Used in treatment of insomnia. Often leaves an 'after-taste'. May cause giddiness, weakness, depression, and 'hangover'. Stimulates its own metabolism. Danger of drug interactions. Coma in overdosage with severe respiratory depression. No antidote. Treated by supportive measures.

Ethinyloestradiol Synthetic female sex hormone with similar actions and adverse effects to **Dienoestrol**. Combined with progestational drug in some oral contraceptives and in treatment of acne and hirsutism.

Ethionamide Anti-tuberculous agent. High incidence of adverse effects, mainly on gastro-intestinal tract.

Ethisterone Similar actions and adverse effects to **Progesterone**.

Ethoglucid Cytotoxic agent. Has been used in the treatment of various malignant conditions. Adverse effects include nausea, baldness, and oedema.

Ethoheptazine Analgesic for mild to moderate pain. Adverse effects include nausea and drowsiness.

Ethomoxane Alpha-adrenoceptor blocking drug similar to **Phentolamine**.

Ethopropazine Parasympatholytic used in treatment of parkinsonism. Less effective than **Benzhexol** and causes more frequent side effects.

Ethosalmide Analgesic, with similar actions and adverse effects to **Salicylamide**.

Ethosuximide Anticonvulsant. Suppresses epileptic discharges in the brain. Used in treatment of petit mal (absence seizures) but not for major epilepsy. May cause nausea and vomiting, drowsiness or excitation, photophobia, and Parkinson-like symptoms. Coma with respiratory depression in overdosage. No antidote. Supportive treatment only.

Ethotoin Anticonvulsant essentially similar to **Phenytoin**, but less toxic and less effective.

Ethyl biscoumacetate Anticoagulant drug, with actions similar to **Warfarin**.

Ethylene diamine Pharmaceutical aid used in manufacture of **Aminophylline** and of some creams for topical application. Can produce allergic dermatitis by both topical and systemic administration.

Ethyl nicotinate Topical vasodilator. See **Nicotinic acid**.

Ethyloestrenol Anabolic steroid. Adverse effects as for **Testosterone**.

Ethyl salicylate Similar to **Methyl salicylate**.

Ethynodiol Similar actions and adverse effects to **Progesterone**. Combined with oestrogenic agent in some oral contraceptives.

Etidronate disodium Used to treat Paget's disease of bone (osteitis deformans). Adverse effects include diarrhoea and nausea.

Etodolac Non-steroid anti-inflammatory/analgesic, with actions and uses similar to **Ibuprofen**. Adverse effects include gastro-intestinal intolerance, but claimed to produce less gastric bleeding than other drugs in this group.

Etomidate Used by injection for induction of anaesthesia. May cause pain on injection, hypotension and involuntary movements.

Etoposide Cytotoxic drug used in treatment of malignant disease. Adverse effects include nausea, vomiting, and bone marrow depression.

Etretinate Synthetic derivative of retinoic acid (**Vitamin A**) used in treatment of severe intractable psoriasis and some other serious disorders of skin growth. Adverse effects include teratogenic actions, dryness of mouth and other mucous membranes, exfoliation of the skin, hair loss, and disorders of liver function and blood fats. Acute overdosage produces severe headache, nausea, vomiting and drowsiness, requiring immediate withdrawal of the drug and non-specific supportive treatment. Contraindicated in pregnancy.

Eucalyptus Essential oil used internally to relieve catarrh and externally as rubefacient.

Eucatropine Parasympatholytic mydriatic similar to **Homatropine**.

F

Factor VIII Blood clotting factor that is deficient in haemophilia and Von Willebrand's disease. Used intravenously to stop episodes of uncontrollable bleeding.

Felypressin Vasoconstrictor polypeptide used in some local anaesthetic preparations. Less likely than sympathomimetic vasoconstrictors to cause cardiac arrhythmias, and does not interact with antidepressant drugs.

Fenbufen Non-steroid anti-inflammatory/analgesic, with action and uses similar to **Ibuprofen**. Has long duration of action and needs only twice daily dosage. Adverse effects include gastro-intestinal intolerance, skin rashes, dizziness and headaches. Contraindicated in hypersensitivity to **Acetylsalicylic acid**.

Fencamfamin CNS stimulant. Adverse effects include anxiety and restlessness.

Fenclofenac Anti-inflammatory/analgesic, with actions, uses, and adverse effects similar to **Ibuprofen**.

Fenfluramine Anti-obesity, with central anorectic and peripheral metabolic effects. May produce diarrhoea, sedation, and sleep disturbance. Contraindicated in patients taking monoamine oxidase inhibitors.

Fennel Essential oil used as carminative.

Fenoprofen Anti-inflammatory/analgesic, with similar actions and uses to **Indomethacin**.

Fenoterol Actions and adverse effects similar to **Salbutamol**.

Fentanyl (c) Narcotic analgesic, with actions and uses similar to **Morphine**. More potent analgesic and respiratory depressant, but shorter action.

Ferric ammonium citrate Actions and adverse effects similar to **Ferrous sulphate**.

Ferric hydroxide Iron salt, with actions similar to **Ferrous sulphate**.

Ferrous fumarate Actions and adverse effects similar to **Ferrous sulphate**.

Ferrous gluconate Actions and adverse effects similar to **Ferrous sulphate**.

Ferrous glycine sulphate See **Ferrous sulphate**.

Ferrous succinate Actions and adverse effects similar to **Ferrous sulphate**.

Ferrous sulphate Used as a source of iron to replenish body iron stores in iron deficiency anaemia. Adverse effects include black faeces, abdominal pain, constipation, and diarrhoea. Liquid formulations can stain teeth black.

Flavoxate Antispasmodic used in bladder disorders. Adverse effects include headache and dry mouth.

Flecainide Antiarrhythmic, with actions and adverse effects similar to **Lignocaine** but active by mouth. Used to treat and prevent life-threatening, irregular cardiac rhythms.

Fluclorolone Topical **Corticosteroid** used in psoriasis and eczema.

Flucloxacillin Antibiotic. Similar properties to **Cloxacillin**, but better absorbed.

Flucytosine Antifungal agent active orally against systemic *Candida* infections. Adverse effects include bone marrow depression.

Fludrocortisone Potent salt-retaining **Corticosteroid** used in adrenal insufficiency. Adverse effects include oedema, hypertension, and electrolyte imbalance.

Flufenamic acid Anti-inflammatory/analgesic essentially similar to **Mefenamic acid**.

Flumethasone Topical **Corticosteroid** used in psoriasis and eczema.

Flunisolide Potent synthetic **Corticosteroid** similar to **Dexamethasone**. Used by nasal spray for treatment of allergic rhinitis.

Flunitrazepam Benzodiazepine hypnotic/anxiolytic with actions, uses, and adverse effects similar to **Nitrazepam**. Recommended only for short-term treatment of insomnia.

Fluocinolone Topical **Corticosteroid** used in psoriasis and eczema.

Fluocinonide Topical **Corticosteroid** used in psoriasis and eczema.

Fluocortolone Topical **Corticosteroid** used in psoriasis and eczema.

Fluorescein Staining agent used for detection of damage to the cornea and as a test of pancreatic function.

Fluorometholone Potent synthetic **corticosteroid**, similar to **Dexamethasone**.

Fluorouracil Cytotoxic, used in the treatment of metastatic cancer of the colon, breast cancer and other solid tumours. May be used topically for some skin lesions. Adverse effects include bone marrow suppression and central nervous system disturbances.

Flupenthixol Tranquillizer, with antidepressant and anxiolytic actions but little sedative effects. Used in depressive and anxiety states associated with inertia and apathy. Adverse effects include restlessness, insomnia, hypotension, and extrapyramidal disturbances. Not recommended for children or excitable patients or in advanced cardiac, renal, or hepatic disease.

Fluphenazine Phenothiazine tranquillizer similar to **Chlorpromazine** but longer acting. Used in treatment of psychoses, confusion, and agitation. Oral treatment required only once a day. Available as a 'depot' intramuscular injection which is active for 10–28 days. Adverse effects similar to **Chlorpromazine** but more frequently causes involuntary movements.

Fluprednylidene Topical **Corticosteroid** used in psoriasis and eczema.

Flurandrenolone Topical **Corticosteroid** used in psoriasis and eczema.

Flurazepam Benzodiazepine tranquillizer/hypnotic. Used in the treatment of insomnia. Essentially similar to **Nitrazepam**.

Flurbiprofen Anti-inflammatory/analgesic, with actions, uses, and adverse effects similar to **Ibuprofen**.

Fluspirilene Tranquillizer used in schizophrenia. Adverse effects include involuntary movements and low blood pressure.

Folic acid Used in folate-deficient megaloblastic anaemias of pregnancy, malnutrition, and malabsorption states. May precipitate neuropathy in untreated **Hydroxocobalamin** deficiency.

Folinic acid Used as an antidote to antifolate cytotoxic agents and in the treatment of megaloblastic anaemias, other than due to vitamin B_{12} **(Hydroxocobalamin)** deficiency.

Formaldehyde As a solution used topically for treatment of warts.

Framycetin Antibiotic derivative of **Neomycin** used topically for skin infections and by mouth for gastro-enteritis and bowel sterilization.

Frangula Mild purgative, with actions, etc. similar to **Cascara**.

Frusemide Potent diuretic which causes greater reduction in sodium reabsorption by the kidney than occurs with the thiazide diuretics (see **Bendrofluazide**. Rapid onset of action when given orally or intravenously. Used in emergency treatment of fluid overload, especially pulmonary oedema and in cases resistant to thiazides. May also be used as antihypertensive. Adverse effects similar to **Bendrofluazide**.

Fuller's earth Adsorbant. Used in poisoning due to the weedkiller paraquat, which it binds strongly. Administered orally or directly into stomach via naso-gastric tube. May be given with **Magnesium sulphate** to promote diarrhoea and thus attempt to empty the gut of paraquat.

Furazolidone Poorly absorbed antibacterial drug used in bacterial diarrhoea and gastro-enteritis. Adverse effects include nausea, vomiting, rashes, haemolysis in predisposed patients, and flushing with alcohol.

Fusafungine Antibiotic administrated by aerosol for infections of upper respiratory tract.

Fusidic acid Steroid antibiotic used for infections by **Penicillin**-resistant staphylococci. Adverse effects include nausea and vomiting.

G

Gallamine Skeletal muscle relaxant used during surgical procedures under general anaesthesia. Has action similar to **Tubocurarine**.

Gamma-benzene hexachloride Applied topically for treatment of lice, scabies, and other infestations. Adverse effects include convulsions if ingested.

Gefarnate Used for treatment of peptic ulcer. May cause skin rashes.

Gelatin Protein used as a nutrient in the preparation of some oral medicines and suppositories, and in a sponge-like form as a haemostatic.

Gemeprost Synthetic prostaglandin which acts on the uterus to prepare it for delivery of the foetus. Used as a pessary to prepare the uterus for surgical termination of pregnancy.

Gentamicin Bactericidal aminoglycoside antibiotic injection with spectrum similar to **Neomycin**, but specially active against *Pseudomonas aeruginosa*. Adverse effects include ototoxicity and nephrotoxicity, particularly in renal failure. Potentiates neuromuscular blockade.

Gestronol Hormone, with similar actions to **Progesterone**.

Glauber's salts See **Sodium sulphate**.

Glibenclamide Oral antidiabetic drug, with actions and uses similar to **Chlorpropamide**.

Glibornuride Oral antidiabetic drug, with actions and uses similar to **Chlorpropamide**.

Gliclazide Oral antidiabetic, with actions, uses, and adverse effects similar to **Chlorpropamide**. Also reduces adhesiveness of blood platelets and thus may reduce the cardiovascular complications of diabetes.

Glipizide Oral antidiabetic drug, with actions and uses similar to **Chlorpropamide**.

Gliquidone Oral antidiabetic, with similar action to **Chlorpropamide** but rapidly metabolized by the liver and excreted in the faeces to give a short duration of effects similar to **Tolbutamide**. Recommended when there is a greater danger of hypoglycaemia (e.g., in the elderly). Adverse effects include gastro-intestinal upsets and skin rashes.

Glucagon Polypeptide hormone produced by alpha-cells of pancreas. Causes increase in blood sugar, release of several other hormones, and increases force of cardiac contraction. Used in tests of carbohydrate metabolism and in treatment of heart failure. May cause nausea and vomiting but cardiac arrhythmias are said not to occur.

Glutaraldehyde As a solution used to treat warts.

Gluten Constituent of wheat starch responsible for bowel disorders in gluten-sensitive individuals. These conditions respond to treatment with a gluten-free diet.

Glutethimide (c) Hypnotic/sedative closely related to the barbiturates. Generalized depressant action on CNS and some anticholinergic effects. Used in treatment of insomnia. May cause 'hangover', blurring of vision, and gastric irritation. As with the barbiturates, tolerance and addiction may occur. Induces its own metabolism with danger of drug interaction. Coma with respiratory depression in overdosage. No antidote. Treatment is supportive.

Glycerin Carbohydrate used as a sweetening agent in some mixtures and pastilles. Used topically in skin preparations for water retaining and softening properties. In suppositories or enemas, it promotes bowel peristalsis and evacuation.

Glycerin suppositories Local lubricant purgative.

Glycerol See **Glycerin**.

Glycerophosphates Used widely in 'tonic' preparations as a source of phosphorus.

Glyceryl trinitrate Vasodilator for symptomatic or prophylactic treatment of angina pectoris. Administered as sublingual tablets or oral spray for rapid absorption at onset of symptoms or applied as gel to skin for sustained absorption in prophylaxis. May also be used intravenously to treat cardiac failure, during hypotensive surgery or during cardiac surgery to prevent myocardial infarction. Adverse effects include headache, dizziness, and flushing. Loses potency if not stored away from light and under cool conditions. Applications to skin may cause local allergic reactions.

Glycine Amino acid used with antacids in gastric hyperacidity, and with aspirin to reduce its gastric irritation.

Glycol salicylate Rubefacient. Essentially similar to **Salicylic acid**.

Glycopyrronium Anticholinergic similar to **Atropine**, used in peptic ulcer, gastric hyperacidity, and to reduce excessive sweating.

Glymidine Oral antidiabetic with actions and uses similar to **Chlorpropamide**.

Gold salts Anti-inflammatory agent, apparently specific for rheumatoid arthritis. Mechanism of action unknown. Given as a course of intramuscular injections. Toxic reactions are common including stomatitis, dermatitis, nausea, vomiting, and diarrhoea. May cause hepatitis, nephritis, and bone marrow depression. Not given if evidence of pre-existing liver or kidney disease.

Gonadorelin Hormone produced in the hypothalamus of the brain which stimulates the ovarian hormones luteinizing hormone (LH) and follicle-stimulating hormone (FSH). Used as pulsatile subcutaneous or intravenous injection for treatment of amenorrhoea and infertility due to ovarian hormone deficiency. May cause gastro-intestinal symptoms, skin rashes, and abdominal pain.

Gonadotrophin Pituitary hormone that stimulates gonadal activity. Used in infertility and delayed puberty.

Gramicidin Antibiotic used by local application to skin, wounds, burns, and nose and mouth infections. Toxic if ingested or injected.

Grindelia Used as expectorant and antispasmodic. Adverse effects include kidney irritation in large doses.

Griseofulvin Antibiotic active against fungal infections of skin and nails when taken orally. May require higher doses in patients on anticonvulsant drugs.

Guaiphenesin Used to reduce sputum viscosity.

Guanethidine Adrenergic neurone blocking drug. Used in hypertension. Eye drops used in glaucoma and hyperthyroid eye signs. Adverse effects include postural hypotension, nasal stuffiness, diarrhoea, fluid retention, and impotence. Action antagonized by tricyclic antidepressants and sympathomimetics (e.g., when used as nasal decongestants in 'cold cures').

Guanochlor Antihypertensive adrenergic neurone blocking drug with actions similar to **Guanethidine**.

Guanoxan Antihypertensive adrenergic neurone blocking drug with actions similar to **Guanethidine**.

Guar Flour See **Guar gum**.

Guar gum Binding agent in tablets, thickening agent in foods. Takes in moisture from the gut and produces feeling of satiety by the bulk thus formed. Used in treatment of obesity and in diabetes mellitus where it may help to stabilize blood glucose levels.

H

Halcinonide Topical **Corticosteroid** used in psoriasis and eczema.

Haloperidol Butyrophenone tranquillizer. Used in treatment of psychosis where it has similar effects to **Chlorpromazine** but more potent. Has anti-emetic action but lacks anticholinergic and alpha-adrenolytic effects. May cause involuntary movements, drowsiness, depression, hypotension, sweating, skin reactions, and jaundice. In overdosage effects and treatment similar to **Chlorpromazine**.

Halopyramine Antihistamine similar to **Promethazine**.

Halothane Potent inhalational anaesthetic used for major surgery. Adverse effects include slowing of the heart and fall in blood pressure. May cause liver damage with jaundice in susceptible patients on repeated exposure.

Heparin Anticoagulant produced in mast cells and obtained from bovine lung. Acts by preventing several reactions in the blood-clotting mechanism. Given by injection only. Used to prevent formation or spread of blood clots as in deep vein thrombosis of the legs or heart valve prostheses. May produce allergic reactions and, on prolonged use, osteoporosis. Heparin-induced haemorrhage may be controlled by **Protamine sulphate**.

Heparinoid See **Heparin**.

Hepatitis B vaccine Vaccine prepared from purified inactivated viral antigens for protection against transmissable viral hepatitis. Used in 'at risk' populations (e.g., health-care personnel and drug abusers). Adverse effects include fever, joint pains, nausea, tiredness, and rashes.

Heptaminol Used as cardiac stimulant in bronchitis.

Heroin (c) See **Diamorphine**.

Hetastarch Polysaccharide used intravenously instead of blood or plasma to maintain blood volume.

Hexachlorophane Topical antiseptic used in soaps, creams, lotions, and dusting powders. Adverse effects include allergy, light sensitivity, and CNS effects if absorbed or ingested.

Hexamethonium Ganglion-blocking drug used parenterally in hypertension. Adverse effects include postural hypotension, dry mouth, paralysis of accommodation, retention of urine, constipation, and impotence.

Hexamine Antiseptic used topically and for urinary infections. For the latter use, the urine must be rendered acid by also giving **Ammonium chloride** which liberates formaldehyde from the hexamine. May cause painful micturition, frequency, and haematuria.

Hexamine mandelate Compound of **Hexamine** and **Mandelic acid**, used as urinary antiseptic. Requires acid urine. Adverse effects include nausea and vomiting.

Hexetidine Topical antibacterial/antifungal/antitrichomonas.

Hexobarbitone (c) Barbiturate hypnotic essentially like **Amylobarbitone**.

Hexylresorcinol Antiworm. Also used as antiseptic agent for throat infections.

Histamine Mediator of many body functions including gastric secretion, inflammatory and allergic responses. Produces skin vasodilation. Used in test of gastric acid production. Adverse effects include headache, hypotension, bronchospasm, and diarrhoea.

Homatropine Parasympatholytic with actions, toxic effects, etc. similar to **Atropine**. Used as a mydriatic because when compared with **Atropine** its action is more rapid, less prolonged, and more easily reversed by **Physostigmine**.

Hyaluronidase Enzyme that assists dispersal and absorption of subcutaneous and intramuscular injections. Hastens resorption of blood and fluid in body cavities. Adverse effects include allergic reactions.

Hydralazine Vasodilator antihypertensive drug. Adverse effects include tachycardia, headache, marrow depression, acute rheumatoid syndrome, and systemic lupus erythematosus syndrome.

Hydrargaphen Mercurial antibacterial/antifungal used topically for skin and ear infections. Adverse effects include allergic reactions.

Hydrochlorothiazide Thiazide diuretic similar to **Bendrofluazide**.

Hydrocortisone Naturally occurring adrenocorticosteroid hormone with similar actions, etc. to **Cortisone**.

Hydroflumethiazide Thiazide diuretic similar to **Bendrofluazide**.

Hydrogen peroxide Disinfectant/deodorant. Acts by rapid but short-lived release of oxygen. Used for cleaning wounds. Also helps to detach dead tissue. Other uses include mouth wash, treatment of acne and minor skin infections, and bleaching hair.

Hydrotalcite Antacid used in peptic ulcer and gastric hyperacidity.

Hydrous wool fat Purified waxy substance obtained from the wool of sheep plus water. Used as a base for ointments. May produce skin sensitization.

Hydroxocobalamin (Vitamin B_{12}) Used for the treatment of pernicious anaemia or specific deficiency states. Parenteral.

Hydroxyapatite Calcium salt used as a source of calcium and phosphorus in osteoporosis, rickets, and osteomalacia.

Hydroxychloroquine Antimalarial agent: see **Chloroquine**.

Hydroxyprogesterone Actions and uses similar to **Progesterone**.

Hydroxyquinoline Topical antibacterial/antifungal deodorant.

Hydroxyurea Cytotoxic agent for oral administration.

Hydroxyzine CNS depressant. Used to relieve tension and anxiety in emotional disturbances but less effective than **Chlorpromazine** and similar tranquillizers in the psychoses. May cause excessive drowsiness, headache, dry mouth, itching, and convulsions. Coma in overdosage. No antidote; supportive treatment only.

Hyoscine butylbromide Parasympatholytic, with peripheral actions similar to **Atropine** but of shorter duration. Used as an antispasmodic similar to **Propantheline** but effective only by injection.

Hyoscine hydrobromide Parasympatholytic, with central and peripheral actions similar to **Atropine** except that it produces central depression and hypnosis rather than stimulation and that it tends to slow the heart. Used for pre-operative medication where the hypnotic effect makes it preferable to atropine and as an anti-emetic for travel sickness. Adverse effects, etc. otherwise as for **Atropine**.

Hyoscine methobromide Similar to **Hyoscine hydrobromide**.

Hyoscyamine See **Atropine**.

Hypromellose Indigestible plant residue similar to **Methylcellulose** but used mainly in eye drops as lubricant (e.g., in so-called artificial tears for dry eyes).

I

Ibuprofen Non-steroid anti-inflammatory/analgesic. Reduces inflammation by inhibition of prostaglandin synthesis which forms part of the inflammatory process. Also inhibits the same enzymes in gastric mucosa. Used in rheumatoid arthritis and other arthritic conditions. Gastro-intestinal symptoms, including blood loss, less common than with **Acetylsalicylic acid**. Headache and other CNS symptoms have been described.

Ichthammol Dermatological preparation, with slight antibacterial effects. Used in creams and ointments for chronic skin conditions.

Idoxuridine Antiviral agent used in local treatment of herpes infections.

Ifosfamide Cytotoxic drug, with uses and adverse effects similar to **Cyclophosphamide**.

Imipramine Antidepressant, blocks neuronal re-uptake of **Noradrenaline, Dopamine**, and 5-hydroxytryptamine. Adverse effects include anticholinergic actions of dry mouth, blurred vision, precipitation of glaucoma, retention of urine, and constipation; also produces cardiac arrhythmias, potentiates direct sympathomimetic pressor amines and antagonizes action of **Guanethidine, Bethanidine, Debrisoquine** and **Clonidine**. Coma, convulsions and cardiac arrhythmias in overdosage. Treatment supportive.

Immunoglobulin G Concentrate of antibodies derived from human plasma. Used to convey short-term immunity to some virus infections including hepatitis A, measles and rubella.

Inactivated lactobacilli Vaccine from bacteria found in the vagina of women suffering from trichomonal infection. The vaccine provokes the immune response to infections including trichomoniasis and thus helps to prevent recurrent infections.

Indapamide Derivative of **Frusemide**, used as antihypertensive in sub-diuretic doses. Larger doses have diuretic action and adverse effects similar to **Bendrofluazide**.

Indomethacin Non-steroid anti-inflammatory/analgesic, used in treatment of inflammatory joint disease. Adverse effects include headache, vertigo, depression, confusion, and gastro-intestinal symptoms including perforation and haemorrhage.

Indoprofen Non-steroid anti-inflammatory/analgesic, with actions, uses, and adverse effects similar to **Ibuprofen**. Recently withdrawn.

Indoramin Alpha-adrenoceptor blocking drug, used in hypertension, peripheral vascular disease, and prophylaxis of migraine. Produces sedation and nasal stuffiness.

Inosine pranobex Antiviral active against herpes simplex in skin and mucous membranes. Does not act directly against the virus, but increases the body's cellular immune response. Metabolized to uric acid and thus may cause elevated uric acid levels. Caution if used in gout or renal failure.

Inositol nicotinate Dilates peripheral blood vessels. Used for chilblains and other conditions where peripheral blood circulation is thought to be poor. Large doses may cause fall in blood pressure and slowing of heart.

Insulin Hormone. Available as pig or beef insulin derived from animal pancreas and as human insulin now available by synthesis from animal insulin or by genetic engineering from bacterial sources. Causes a fall in blood sugar levels and increased storage of glycogen in the liver. Used parenterally to treat diabetes. Different formulations are produced to provide varied duration of action. Adverse effects include hypoglycaemia and subcutaneous fat atrophy.

Iodine Halogen, converted to iodide in the body and used in production of thyroid hormone. Low dietary intake leads to reduced thyroid function (myxoedema). Large doses may be given by mouth to suppress thyroid function prior to surgical removal of thyroid tissue when the gland is over-active. May cause hypersensitivity with headache, laryngitis, bronchitis, and rashes. May also be used on the skin as a disinfectant.

Ipecacuanha Plant extract used in small doses as an expectorant in cough mixtures. Emetic effect if larger doses (syrup of ipecacuanha) are used in children as emergency treatment of ingested poisons.

Ipratropium Anticholinergic used by inhalation for its bronchodilator action in chronic bronchitis and asthma. Adverse effects similar to **Atropine**, but much reduced when given by inhalation and are seen only at high doses.

Iprindole Antidepressant, with actions, uses, and adverse effects similar to **Imipramine**.

Iproniazid Monoamine oxidase inhibitor/antidepressant. Actions, uses, and adverse effects as for **Phenelzine**.

Iron dextran injection Parenteral formulation for iron-deficiency anaemia. Adverse effects include pain on injection, skin staining, vomiting, headache, and dizziness. Anaphylactic reactions may accompany intravenous infusion particularly.

Iron sorbitol injection Intramuscular formulation for iron deficiency anaemia. Adverse effects as for **Iron dextran injection**.

Isoaminile citrate Cough suppressant used on its own or in cough linctus. No analgesic or sedative effects. Does not depress respiration. May cause dizziness, nausea, and constipation or diarrhoea.

Isocarboxazid Monoamine oxidase inhibitor/antidepressant. Actions, uses, and adverse effects as for **Phenelzine**.

Isoconazole Used to treat fungal and protozoal vaginal infections. Actions and adverse effects similar to **Metronidazole**.

Isoetharine Bronchodilator. Actions, uses, and adverse effects as for **Salbutamol**.

Isoflurane Potent inhalational anaesthetic used for major surgery. Has also analgesic properties. More potent than **Halothane** in depressing respiration and enhancing effects of muscle relaxants (e.g., **Tubocurarine**) but less likely to sensitize the heart to catecholamines.

Isometheptene Sympathomimetic agent, with actions and adverse effects similar to **Adrenaline**. Used in symptomatic treatment of migraine where it is said to constrict the dilated blood vessels that cause the throbbing headache.

Isoniazid Synthetic anti-tuberculous agent. About 60 percent of Caucasians are slow inactivators by acetylation, genetically determined. Adverse effects include peripheral neuropathy, pellagra, mental disturbances, and convulsions, which may be reduced by administration of **Pyridoxine**.

Isoprenaline Beta-adrenoceptor agonist used in bronchial asthma by inhalation or orally. Adverse effects include tachycardia, arrhythmias, and tremor. May also be used as intravenous infusion in treatment of shock. More likely to cause cardiac arrhythmias than **Dopamine** or **Dobutamine**.

Isopropamide Anticholinergic with actions and adverse effects similar to **Atropine**. Used in treatment of gastro-intestinal colic, peptic ulceration, and as a decongestant in symptomatic relief of the common cold.

Isosorbide mononitrate Vasodilator used for prophylaxis of angina. An active metabolite of **Isosorbide dinitrate**, it is not metabolized further and may thus have a more predictable effect. Adverse effects are similar to **Glyceryl trinitrate**.

Isosorbide dinitrate (Sorbide nitrate) Dilates blood vessels. Similar actions and adverse effects to **Glyceryl trinitrate** but longer action. Used for symptomatic and prophylactic treatment of angina and in resistant heart failure.

Isotretinoin Vitamin A derivative, used to treat severe acne not responsive to antibiotic therapy. Thought to act directly on sebaceous glands in the skin to reduce sebum production. Adverse effects include dryness of skin, mucous membranes and conjunctivae. Teratogenesis, nausea, headache, malaise, joint pains, hair loss, and biochemical evidence of liver damage may also occur. Contraindicated in the presence of liver or kidney disease and in pregnancy.

Isoxsuprine Beta-adrenoceptor agonist, produces uterine relaxation. Used in premature labour. Adverse effects include tachycardia, cardiac arrhythmias, and tremor.

Ispaghula Purgative. Dried, ripe seeds of *Plantago ovata*. Increases faecal bulk. Mechanism of action similar to that of **Methylcellulose**.

Ispaghula husk As for **Ispaghula**, but contains only outer layers of dried seeds and is more potent than whole seeds.

K

Kanamycin Bactericidal aminoglycoside antibiotic with actions and spectrum similar to **Neomycin**, but less ototoxic. Used in gram-negative septicaemia, with monitoring of blood levels, particularly in renal failure. Potentiates neuromuscular blockade.

Kaolin Adsorbant. Used externally as a dusting powder and by mouth as treatment for diarrhoea where it increases faecal bulk and slows passage through the gut. Once thought to have specific adsorbent effect for poisonous substances but it is now known that the adsorbent effect is a general one.

Ketamine Parenteral anaesthetic with analgesic properties in subanaesthetic doses. Rapid onset of action, but may cause psychotic symptoms, including hallucinations, the frequency of which can be reduced by giving **Diazepam** or **Droperidol**. Contraindicated in patients with high blood pressure or known psychosis.

Ketazolam Benzodiazepine anxiolytic, with actions and adverse effects similar to **Diazepam**. Presently used to treat anxiety and muscle spasms.

Ketoconazole Used to treat internal and external fungal infections. Adverse effects include nausea, rashes, and jaundice.

Ketoprofen Anti-inflammatory/analgesic, with actions, uses and adverse effects similar to **Ibuprofen**.

Ketotifen Preventative treatment for asthma. Has the actions of an antihistamine, similar to **Promethazine** and also blocks allergic mechanisms by a mechanism similar to **Sodium cromoglycate**. Adverse effects include dry mouth, dizziness, and sedation.

L

Labetalol Antihypertensive. Has both alpha and beta-adrenoceptor blocking actions. Uses and adverse effects similar to **Propranolol**. Postural hypotension may occur.

Lactic acid Used intravenously as dilute solution in treatment of acidosis. Acts less rapidly than **Sodium bicarbonate**. Also used topically as strong solutions in treatment of warts.

Lachesine Parasympatholytic, similar to **Tropicamide**. Used in the eye as a mydriatic and cycloplegic.

Lactulose Purgative. A synthetic disaccharide (galactose plus fructose) that is not absorbed but broken down by gut bacteria to nonabsorbable anions that increase the faecal mass by osmotic effects. Effective but expensive. Has been recommended for use in liver failure to reduce absorption of ammonia from the gut.

Laevodopa See **Levodopa**.

Laevulose Carbohydrate. Used intravenously as a source of calories when oral feeding is not possible. In renal failure it is better tolerated than dextrose. Accelerates metabolism of ethyl alcohol and may be used to treat alcohol poisoning. May cause facial flushing, abdominal pain, and localized thrombophlebitis.

Lanatoside C Foxglove derivative with actions, etc. similar to **Digoxin**.

Lanolin Purified, fat-like substance from the wool of sheep. Used in creams for topical use, it is not absorbed but aids the absorption of drugs carried in the cream. Otherwise used for its emulsifying effect in bland creams and cosmetics. May cause skin sensitization.

L-Asparaginase (Colaspase) Cytotoxic enzyme derived from bacterial culture; used in neoplastic disease. Adverse effects include nausea, vomiting, pyrexia, neurotoxicity, hypersensitivity reactions, and bone marrow depression.

Latamoxef Injectable, broad-spectrum antibiotic structurally related to

Penicillins and **Cephalosporins** but active against wider range of organisms. Adverse effects include rashes and gastro-intestinal symptoms.

L-Dopa See **Levodopa**.

Lecithins Phospholipids found in both animal and vegetable foods. Used as emulsifying and stabilizing agents in skin preparations.

Leucinocaine See **Panthesine**.

Levallorphan Narcotic antagonist similar to **Nalorphine**. Less likely to cause severe withdrawal symptoms in 'addicts'.

Levamisole Antiworm treatment. Used mainly in veterinary practice but also in man against *Ascaris* sp. (roundworm). Adverse effects include nausea, vomiting, abdominal pain, and fall in blood pressure.

Levodopa Amino acid. Converted in body to **Dopamine**, a neurotransmitter substance that is deficient in Parkinson's disease. Controls rigidity and improves movements but less effect on tremor than anticholinergic drugs (e.g., **Benzhexol**). May cause gastro-intestinal symptoms, hypotension, involuntary movements, and psychiatric disturbances. Side effects may be reduced by combination with peripheral inhibitors of dopamine synthesis (e.g., **Carbidopa**). Contraindicated/caution in cardiovascular disease and psychiatric disturbance. Effects diminished by phenothiazines (e.g., **Chlorpromazine**), **Methyldopa, Reserpine, Pyridoxine**.

Levonorgestrel See Norgestrel.

Levorphanol (c) Narcotic analgesic similar to **Morphine**, but more reliable when given by mouth. Useful in the management of severe chronic pain in terminal disease.

Lidoflazine Preventive treatment for angina. Increases blood supply to heart by dilating the blood vessels of the heart without increasing oxygen consumption. May cause gastric disturbance and dizziness.

Lignocaine Local anaesthetic/antiarrhythmic. Stabilizes nerve cell membranes to prevent impulse conduction. Used topically or by injection for local anaesthesia in minor operations. Intravenous injection or infusion used to treat abnormal heart rhythms. Excessive doses also block motor impulses and normal cardiac conduction. May cause hypotension, CNS depression and convulsions. Metabolized by liver and therefore used with caution in liver disease. Short action prevents use as oral antiarrhythmic.

Lincomycin Antibiotic active against **Penicillin**-resistant staphylococci and bacteroides. Adverse effects include rashes, diarrhoea, and pseudomembranous colitis.

Lindane Organochlorine insecticide. Used topically on skin/hair for lice and scabies. Safe, providing not ingested, but emergence of resistance strains of the parasites limits its effectiveness.

Liothyronine Thyroid hormone, probably the active hormone to which **Thyroxine** is converted. Given by mouth or injection it has effects similar to **Thyroxine** but more rapid and short-lived. Used when rapid effect is needed (e.g., in myxoedema coma). Used with care if there is evidence of cardiovascular disease as it may precipitate cardiac failure.

Liquid paraffin Purgative. Lubricates faecal material in colon and rectum. Used when straining is undesirable or defaecation painful (e.g., after operations for haemorrhoids). Reduces absorption of fat-soluble **Vitamin A** and **Vitamin D**, and in chronic use can cause paraffinomas in mesenteric lymph glands. May leak from anal sphincter. Also used in some topical skin and eye preparations as a lubricant and an aid to removal of crusts.

Liquorice Dried plant root with expectorant and mild anti-inflammatory properties. Used as a flavouring/expectorant in cough mixtures. **Deglycyrrhizinised** liquorice is used in treatment of peptic ulceration. Large doses may cause salt and water retention leading to hypertension and /or cardiac failure.

Lithium salts Usually given as carbonate or citrate, provides lithium ions which substitute for sodium in excitable tissues and reduce brain catecholamine levels. Used in prophylactic treatment of mania and depression. Caution in cardiac or renal disease. Needs careful control of plasma levels. Adverse effects include tremor, vomiting, diarrhoea, ataxia, blurred vision, thirst, polyuria leading to confusion and fits, and coma in gross overdosage. Lithium excretion may be enhanced by forced alkaline diuresis, peritoneal dialysis, or haemodialysis. Intoxication may be precipitated by diuretic therapy or salt restriction.

Liver extracts Extracts of liver prepared for oral use were used for treatment of pernicious anaemia. Unpalatable and irregularly absorbed. Now replaced by the pure vitamin B_{12} (**Hydroxocobalamin**).

Lofepramine Antidepressant, metabolized to **Desipramine** after absorption. Actions, uses, and adverse effects similar to **Amitriptyline**.

Lomustine (CCNU) Cytotoxic drug used in neoplastic disease. Adverse effects include loss of appetite, nausea, vomiting, liver toxicity, and bone marrow depression.

Loperamide Antidiarrhoeal, with actions, uses, and adverse effects similar to **Diphenoxylate**.

Loprazolam Benzodiazepine, used for short-term treatment of insomnia. Actions and adverse effects similar to **Diazepam**.

Lorazepam Benzodiazepine anxiolytic similar to **Diazepam**.

Lormetazepam Benzodiazepine tranquillizer/hypnotic similar to **Nitrazepam**.

LSD (Lysergic acid diethylamide). See **Lysergide**.

Lymecycline Bacteriostatic antibiotic, with actions, adverse effects, and interactions similar to **Tetracycline**.

Lynoestrenol Sex hormone (progestogen) with actions, uses, and adverse effects similar to **Norethisterone**.

Lypressin Hormone extract from posterior pituitary gland of pigs. Actions, uses, and adverse effects similar to **Vasopressin**.

Lysergide Hallucinogen. Not used therapeutically but abused for its psychedelic effects – notably altered visual perception. Consciousness and awareness not altered, but may cause thought disorders, personality changes and apparent psychotic disease. Other 'unwanted' effects include gastro-intestinal disturbance, sweating, and incoordination.

M

Mafenide Sulphonamide antibacterial with actions similar to **Sulphadimidine**. Used topically on skin and as eye drops.

Magaldrate Antacid. Complex hydrated form of **Magnesium sulphate** and aluminium sulphate.

Magnesium antacids Range of magnesium salts used alone or complexed with other compounds. Neutralize gastric acid in treatment of peptic ulceration. Large doses have laxative effect which may be reduced by combination with **Aluminium antacids**. Very little absorbed but danger of toxic magnesium blood levels in renal failure. May reduce absorption of other drugs (e.g., **Tetracyclines**).

Magnesium carbonate Nonsystemic antacid with similar actions, uses, and adverse effects to **Magnesium hydroxide**. Releases carbon dioxide in stomach and may cause belching.

Magnesium citrate Solution used to aid removal or prevent formation of crystals in long-term urinary catheterization.

Magnesium hydroxide Nonsystemic antacid (only 10 percent absorbed). Used in treatment of peptic ulceration. Neutralizes gastric acid and acts longer than **Sodium bicarbonate**. May have laxative effect, which can be prevented by simultaneous use of **Aluminium antacids**.

Magnesium oxide Nonsystemic antacid. Converted to **Magnesium hydroxide** in the stomach and has similar actions and adverse effects.

Magnesium sulphate (Epsom salts) Saline purgative. Absorbed only slowly from gut. Magnesium and sulphate ions attract or retain water by osmosis and thus increase bulk of intestinal contents. Effective in three to six hours. Produces semi-fluid or watery stools, therefore useful as single treatment but not for repeated dosage. Danger of systemic toxicity from magnesium in patients with reduced renal function.

Magnesium trisilicate Nonsystemic antacid used in treatment of peptic ulceration. Neutralization of acid is slow in onset but relatively prolonged due to adsorbent properties of silicic acid formed in the stomach. Has a laxative effect in larger doses. Danger of magnesium toxicity in patients with renal failure.

Malathion Organophosphorus insecticide. Acts by inhibition of cholinesterase and may therefore produce toxic effects due to accumulation of excess **Acetylcholine**. One of the least toxic of this group of insecticides, low concentrations of malathion may be used on human skin for infestation (e.g., lice) without systemic effects. Toxic effects may be treated by antidotes **Atropine** and **Pralidoxime**.

Malic acid Found in apples and pears. Formerly used in tooth-cleaning tablets. Used as part of an astringent skin treatment.

Mandelic acid Excreted unchanged in the urine where it has antibacterial (bacteriostatic) actions. Used orally in combination with **Hexamine** as **Hexamine mandelate**. May also be instilled directly into the bladder during prolonged use of urinary catheters.

Manganese sulphate Occasionally used as a haematinic. Said to increase the effect of **Ferrous sulphate** in treatment of iron-deficiency anaemia.

Mannitol Osmotic diuretic. Opposes reabsorption of water which normally accompanies sodium reabsorption from kidney tubule. Used when there is danger of renal failure (e.g., shock, cardiovascular surgery) and in fluid overload refractory to other diuretics. May cause cardiac failure owing to increased circulating blood volume.

Maprotiline Antidepressant, with actions, uses, and adverse effects similar to **Imipramine**.

Mazindol (c) Anorectic indole derivative with central stimulant properties. Produces tachycardia and rise in blood pressure.

Measles vaccine Live attenuated measles virus for measles immunization. Adverse effects include mild fever, rash, and rare neurological disorders. Use with care if there is a history of convulsions or epilepsy.

Mebendazole Used in treatment of roundworm. Actions and adverse effects as for **Thiabendazole**.

Mebeverine Antispasmodic, with direct action on colonic smooth muscle but no systemic anticholinergic effects. Used for relief of abdominal pain and cramps (e.g., due to irritable colon or non-specific diarrhoea).

Mebhydroline Antihistamine, with uses and adverse effects similar to **Promethazine** but shorter duration of action and less likely to cause sedation.

Mecamylamine Ganglion-blocking drug. Use and adverse effects as for **Hexamethonium**.

Mecillinam Antibiotic for injection. Acts by inhibition of bacterial cell wall synthesis but mechanism of action is different from that of **Penicillins** and **Cephalosporins** such that combination with another drug from these groups may have an enhanced effect. Indicated for serious infections of the urinary and gastro-intestinal tracts. Adverse reactions include skin rashes and cross-sensitivity with **Penicillins** and **Cephalosporins**.

Meclozine Antihistamine, with similar actions, uses, and adverse effects to **Promethazine**.

Medazepam Benzodiazepine anxiolytic similar to **Diazepam** but with less anticonvulsant activity. Used in the treatment of anxiety.

Medigoxin Actions, uses, and adverse effects similar to **Digoxin**.

Medium-chain triglycerides A mixture of triglycerides from straight-chain fatty acids for use in fat malabsorption syndromes.

Medroxyprogesterone Sex hormone, with actions and adverse effects similar to **Progesterone**. Used to treat hormone-dependent malignancies (e.g., of breast, endometrium and prostrate).

Mefenamic acid Anti-inflammatory/analgesic. Mode of action uncertain. Used in treatment of arthritis. May cause severe diarrhoea. Other adverse effects include gastro-intestinal bleeding, exacerbation of asthma, haemolytic anaemia, and bone marrow depression. May enhance action of oral anticoagulants (e.g., **Warfarin**).

Mefruside Diuretic essentially similar to **Bendrofluazide**.

Megestrol Sex hormone, with actions and effects similar to **Progesterone**. Used to suppress **Oestrogen**-dependent tumours of the breast and the uterus by interfering with uptake of oestrogen into the tumour. Adverse effects include weight gain, nausea, skin rashes, hair loss, deep venous thromboses in the legs.

Melphalan Cytotoxic drug used in myelomatosis. Actions and adverse effects similar to **Chlorambucil**.

Menadiol Orally active form of **Vitamin K**.

Menaphthone See **Vitamin K**.

Menotrophin Preparation of follicle-stimulating hormone, derived from human post-menopausal urine, which also possesses some luteinizing hormone activity. Used to stimulate ovulation.

Menthol Aromatic oil used as inhalation, orally as pastilles for relief of respiratory symptoms, or topically on skin where it causes dilatation of blood vessels producing a sense of coldness and analgesia.

Mepenzolate Anticholinergic, with actions and adverse effects similar to **Atropine**. Marked effect upon spasm of colon. Used to relieve pain, distension, and diarrhoea associated with gastro-intestinal disorders.

Mepivacaine Local anaesthetic with actions, adverse effects, and uses similar to **Lignocaine** but not used to treat abnormal heart rhythms.

Meprobamate Minor tranquillizer (anxiolytic) with selective action on hypothalamus and spinal cord. Used in treatment of neuroses, alcoholism, and functional disorders, such as tension headache. May cause gastro-intestinal disorders, headache, dizziness with hypotension, lowered tolerance to alcohol, and withdrawal symptoms. Induces hepatic drug metabolism with danger of drug interactions. Coma with respiratory depression in overdosage. No antidote. Forced alkaline diuresis and haemodialysis may be effective.

Meptazinol Analgesic with narcotic antagonist activity. Actions, uses, and adverse effects similar to **Pentazocine**, but central adverse effects and dependence appear to be less.

Mepyramine Antihistamine, with similar uses and adverse effects to **Promethazine**, but has shorter duration of action and is less likely to cause sedation.

Mequitazine Antihistamine with actions and adverse effects similar to **Promethazine**. Used in treatment of allergic conditions.

Mercaptopurine Cytotoxic drug, inhibiting nucleoprotein synthesis, used in neoplastic disease, particularly leukaemia. Adverse effects include bone marrow depression.

Mersalyl Organic mercurial diuretic. Depresses active reabsorption of sodium and chloride by kidney tubules. Used in treatment of fluid retention. Long-acting; must be administered by intramuscular injection. Danger of excessive loss of sodium and chloride. May cause gastro-intestinal disturbance, skin rashes, and, after prolonged use, kidney damage.

Mesalazine (5-Aminosalicylic acid) Active constituent of **Sulphasalazine**. Used in ulcerative colitis. Free of sulphonamide adverse effects.

Mesna Used to protect the bladder mucosa from the irritant effect upon it of **Cyclophosphamide** and **Ifosfamide**. Acts by combining with their toxic metabolite acrolein. Does not prevent their other toxic effects.

Mesterolone Sex hormone, with actions, uses, and adverse effects similar to **Testosterone**.

Mestranol Sex hormone, with actions, uses, and adverse effects similar to **Oestradiol**.

Metaraminol Sympathomimetic agent with alpha and beta-effects similar to **Adrenaline**. Alpha-effects predominate and thus it has been used to raise blood pressure in hypotension after myocardial infarction. May cause headache, dizziness, nausea, vomiting, and tremor.

Metformin Oral antidiabetic. Increases use of glucose by peripheral tissues. Used alone or in combination with sulphonylureas (e.g., **Chlorpropamide**) or **Insulin**. Most useful in overweight subjects, where it suppresses appetite. May cause nausea, vomiting, and diarrhoea.

Methacholine Parasympathomimetic drug, with muscarinic actions of **Acetylcholine**.

Methacycline Antibacterial, with actions, uses, and adverse effects similar to **Tetracycline**.

Methadone (c) Synthetic narcotic analgesic. Actions similar to **Morphine**, but less sedation, euphoria, and respiratory depression. Used in control of withdrawal symptoms from narcotic addiction and for relief of chronic pain in terminal disease. **Naloxone** is a pure antagonist.

Methallenestril Sex hormone, with actions, uses, and adverse effects similar to **Oestradiol**.

Methaqualone (c) Hypnotic/sedative. General depressant action on CNS. Used in treatment of insomnia. Frequently has 'hangover' effect. May also cause localized loss of sensation with numbness and tingling, as well as skin rashes and gastro-intestinal disturbance. Liable to abuse for so-called 'aphrodisiac' qualities and euphoriant effects. In overdose causes respiratory depression with increased muscle tone and increased reflexes. No antidote. Treatment is supportive.

Methicillin Antibiotic. Similar properties to **Cloxacillin**, but only active parenterally.

Methionine Amino acid, essential constituent of diet. May be used as an antidote in severe poisoning due to **Paracetamol** where it is thought to prevent liver damage by reducing the concentration of a toxic metabolite. Given orally it causes few side effects, principally nausea. Must not be given more than ten hours after the overdose as it may then exacerbate liver damage.

Methixene Parasympatholytic used in treatment of parkinsonism. Actions, etc. similar to **Benzhexol**, but greater effect in reducing tremor.

Methocarbamol Muscle relaxant, with actions, uses, and adverse effects similar to **Mephenesin**.

Methohexitone Ultra-short-acting barbiturate hypnotic. Used for induction of anaesthesia. Actions and adverse effects similar to **Thiopentone sodium**.

Methoserpidine Antihypertensive. Actions, uses, and adverse effects similar to **Reserpine**.

Methotrexate Cytotoxic drug, antagonizing folic acid, used in neoplastic disease, particularly leukaemia. Adverse effects include alopecia, stomatitis, liver toxicity, folate-deficient anaemia, and bone marrow depression.

Methotrimeprazine Antipsychotic, with actions, uses, and adverse effects similar to **Chlorpromazine**.

Methoxamine Sympathomimetic. Stimulates alpha-adrenoceptors to cause constriction of blood vessels and rise in blood pressure. Used to reverse hypotension during anaesthesia. May cause pronounced slowing of heart rate and excessive rise in blood pressure.

Methoxyphenamine Sympathomimetic amine, with predominantly beta-effects. Used for prevention of asthma. Adverse effects include tachycardia, tremor, nausea, and insomnia.

5-Methoxypsoralen Sun screen. Used topically to filter out harmful sun rays. May cause photosensitivity and has been suspected of increasing the incidence of skin cancer.

Methylcellulose Indigestible plant residue used as a lubricating agent in pharmaceutical preparations and as a purgative. Adsorbs water, increases faecal bulk and thus promotes bowel movements. Slow action (0.5–3 days). No important systemic effects.

Methylclothiazide Diuretic essentially similar to **Bendrofluazide**.

Methylcysteine Mucolytic, with actions, uses, and adverse effects similar to **Acetylcysteine**. Used orally as well as by aerosol inhalation.

Methyldopa Antihypertensive. Reduces sympathetic tone by central and peripheral mechanisms. Adverse effects include sedation, depression, nasal stuffiness, fluid retention, impotence, and haemolytic anaemia.

Methylephedrine Sympathomimetic agent, with actions, uses, and adverse effects similar to **Ephedrine**.

Methyl nicotinate Vasodilator/rubefacient used in ointments and creams for topical application at sites of muscle pains in rheumatic conditions (e.g., fibrositis, muscular rheumatism).

Methylpentynol Tertiary alcohol. Hypnotic/sedative. Rapid but short-lived generalized depression of the CNS. Used in treatment of insomnia and anxiety. May cause repeated belching. In overdosage, symptoms resemble inebriation with alcohol. No antidote. Supportive treatment is adequate.

Methylphenobarbitone (c) Anticonvulsant/sedative essentially similar to **Phenobarbitone**.

Methylprednisolone **Corticosteroid**, with actions, uses, and adverse effects similar to **Prednisone**.

Methyl salicylate Rubefacient used for relief of musculo-skeletal pain. Has similar actions and adverse effects to **Acetylsalicylic acid** but not used systemically.

Methyltestosterone Sex hormone, with actions, uses and adverse effects similar to **Testosterone**.

Methyprylone (c) Hypnotic sedative. Related to **Glutethimide** and essentially similar to that drug and **Amylobarbitone**.

Methysergide Serotonin antagonist used in preventive treatment for severe migraine. May cause nausea, abdominal cramp, dizziness, and psychiatric disturbance. Prolonged use may cause retroperitoneal fibrosis resulting in impairment of renal function.

Metirosine Antihypertensive. Enzyme inhibitor which blocks the synthesis of catecholamines by the adrenal gland. Used to control hypertension caused by the adrenal tumour phaeochromocytoma where the raised blood pressure is caused by excess production of catecholamines. Adverse effects include sedation, diarrhoea, and hypersensitivity.

Metoclopramide Anti-emetic with dopamine antagonist actions in brain and peripheral effects on gastro-intestinal tract where it stimulates motility to improve gastric emptying and intestinal transit. May cause drowsiness and involuntary movements. Used to treat nausea and vomiting from most causes and as an adjunct to X-ray examination of the gut.

Metolazone Diuretic essentially similar to **Bendrofluazide**.

Metoprolol Beta-adrenoceptor blocking drug, with limited cardio-selectivity. Uses, side effects, etc. as for **Propranolol**.

Metriphonate Organophosphorus cholinesterase inhibitor, used as an anti-infective in treatment of schistosomiasis. Active only against *S. haematobium*. May cause unwanted cholinergic symptoms as from **Acetylcholine**.

Metronidazole Antimicrobial. Effective against trichomonas, Vincent's organisms, anaerobic bacteria, giardiasis, and amoebiasis. Adverse effects include nausea, metallic taste in mouth, hypersensitivity reactions, **Disulfiram**-like reaction with alcohol.

Metyrapone Inhibits enzyme responsible for synthesis of adrenocorticosteroids. Used in tests of pituitary gland function. May cause gastro-intestinal disturbance and dizziness.

Mexenone Absorbs ultraviolet light and protects skin from sunburn.

Mexiletine Cardiac antiarrhythmic agent similar to **Lignocaine**, but also effective when given by mouth. May cause nausea, vomiting, drowsiness, tremors, convulsions, hypotension, and bradycardia.

Mezlocillin Injectable **Penicillin** antibiotic with broad spectrum of activity against gram-negative bacteria, notably *Pseudomonas* and *Proteus*. Not effective against penicillinase-producing bacteria. Adverse effects as for **Benzylpenicillin**.

Mianserin Antidepressant, with uses similar to **Imipramine**, but without its peripheral autonomic adverse effects.

Miconazole Antifungal agent used topically for skin infections.

Midazolam Intravenous benzodiazepine anxiolytic/sedative, with short duration of action. Used for induction of anaesthesia before minor surgery. Actions and adverse effects similar to **Diazepam**.

Mineral oil See **Liquid paraffin**.

Minocycline Antibacterial, with actions, uses, and adverse effects similar to **Tetracycline**.

Minoxidil Vasodilator/antihypertensive. Reduces muscle tone in peripheral blood vessels. Fluid retention and tachycardia accompany this effect but can be controlled by using concomitant therapy with a diuretic (e.g., **Bendrofluazide**) and a beta-adrenoceptor blocker (e.g., **Propranolol**). Other adverse effects include increased hair growth and breast tenderness. Used mainly in severe hypertension when other drugs fail.

Mistletoe Plant extract, with vasodilator action, Has been recommended for treatment of hypertension and included in mixture for relief of broncho-spasm.

Mithramycin Cytotoxic antibiotic. No longer used to treat cancer itself, but may be used as emergency therapy to reduce hypercalcaemia due to malignant disease. More effective than chelating agents such as **Tri-sodium edetate**, but causes suppression of bone marrow and cannot be used for more than a few days.

Mitrobronitol Cytotoxic drug, with actions, uses, and adverse effects similar to **Busulphan**.

Mitomycin Cytotoxic antibiotic. Used to treat upper gastro-intestinal and breast cancers. Causes delayed effects on the bone marrow, lung fibrosis, and renal damage. Used at six-week intervals to reduce these effects.

Mitozantrone Cytotoxic drug, with actions against resting-phase tumour, as well as those undergoing DNA synthesis. May thus be effective in both slow and rapid growing tumours. Used in advanced breast cancer. May cause bone marrow suppression, hair loss, gastro-intestinal disturbances, heart failure and impaired liver function.

Monosulfiram Parasiticide used topically for treatment of fleas, lice, ticks, and mites. May cause skin rashes. Related to **Disulfiram** and may have similar effects if ingested.

Morazone Analgesic/anti-inflammatory agent. Used only in a compound preparation.

Morphine (c) Poppy derivative. Centrally acting narcotic analgesic used for relief of severe pain. Other potentially useful effects include euphoria and cough suppression. Adverse effects include respiratory depression, nausea, vomiting, constipation, hypotension, physical dependence, and ('addiction') abuse. Coma with danger of death in overdosage. **Naloxone** is a specific antagonist.

Mupirocin Antibiotic, previously known as pseudomonic acid. Used as an ointment to treat bacterial skin infections. Inactive orally.

Mustine hydrochloride (Nitrogen mustard) Cytotoxic drug used in neo-plastic disease. Adverse effects include nausea, vomiting, and bone marrow depression.

N

Nabilone Derivative of cannabis, with anti-emetic and anxiolytic properties. Acts on opiate receptors in the brain to block transmission of vomiting impulses. Used to suppress nausea and vomiting from cytotoxic drugs. Adverse effects include drowsiness, postural hypotension, headaches, tremors, psychosis, and abdominal cramps.

Nadolol Beta-adrenoceptor blocking drug. Uses and adverse effects as for **Propranolol**.

Naftidrofuryl Peripheral vasodilator said to improve cellular metabolism and to relax muscle cells in blood vessel walls. Recommended for treatment of reduced peripheral blood circulation and dementia caused by reduced blood flow. May cause headache, insomnia, and gastro-intestinal disturbance.

Nalbuphine Narcotic analgesic, with agonist and antagonist properties. Uses and adverse effects similar to **Pentazocine**.

Nalidixic acid Urinary antiseptic to which resistance readily occurs. May cause gastro-intestinal symptoms and allergic reactions. May exacerbate epilepsy and respiratory depression.

Nalorphine Narcotic antagonist. Reverses effects of **Morphine** and other narcotic analgesics but less specific than **Naloxone** as has some narcotic activity of its own. Used for reversal of narcotic effects but not when due to **Pentazocine**. May cause hallucinations and thought disturbances. In 'addicts', causes severe withdrawal symptoms.

Naloxone Narcotic antagonist. A true antidote to **Morphine** and other narcotic analgesics. Has no narcotic activity in its own right. Used for reversal of narcotic effects from any narcotic drug especially respiratory depression. Danger of severe withdrawal symptoms if given to those physically dependent ('addicted') on narcotics.

Nandrolone Sex hormone, with actions and adverse effects similar to **Testosterone**, but anabolic effects greater than androgenic effects. Used in treatment of debilitating illness and carcinoma of the breast. Injection only; not active by mouth.

Naphazoline Sympathomimetic agent with marked alpha-adrenergic activity. Used topically on nasal mucosa where its vasoconstrictor effect leads to reduced secretion and mucosal swelling (e.g., in allergic rhinitis). Prolonged use may lead to rebound nasal congestion and secretion. Not used systemically but oral overdosage would cause depression of nervous system and coma.

Naproxen Anti-inflammatory/analgesic, with actions, uses, and adverse effects similar to **Ibuprofen**.

Natamycin Antifungal used topically for fungal infections of the vagina and skin. Not used orally because poorly absorbed and causes gastric irritation. May cause skin rashes.

Nefopam Centrally acting analgesic; mode of action unknown, but not related to the narcotics. Used for acute and chronic pain. Adverse effects include gastro-intestinal upsets, palpitations, and CNS stimulation with nervousness, insomnia, headache, blurred vision, and sweating. Drowsiness is sometimes seen, but respiratory depression and habituation do not occur. Contraindicated in patients with epilepsy, glaucoma, or urinary retention.

Neomycin Bactericidal aminoglycoside antibiotic with spectrum similar to **Streptomycin**, but more active against *Staphylococcus* and *Proteus*. Not used systemically because of risk of ototoxicity and nephrotoxicity. Used topically and orally for bowel sterilization and in liver failure. May cause malabsorption if given for long period. Potentiates neuromuscular blockade.

Neostigmine (Prostigmine) Anticholinesterase with actions similar to **Physostigmine**.

Netilmicin Aminoglycoside antibiotic, with actions, uses, and adverse effects similar to **Gentamicin**.

Niacinamide Vitamin: see **Nicotinic acid**.

Nialamide Antidepressant/monoamine oxidase inhibitor with actions, uses, and adverse effects similar to **Phenelzine**.

Niclosamide Used in treatment of tapeworms. Adverse effects are uncommon as it is not absorbed from the intestinal tract.

Nicofuranose See **Tetranicotinoylfructose**.

Nicotinamide Vitamin: see **Nicotinic acid**.

Nicotinic acid (Vitamin B_7) Vitamin. Deficiency causes pellagra, with dermatitis, diarrhoea, and dementia. Has direct relaxant effect on muscle in peripheral blood vessels and has been used to treat reduced peripheral circulation. Large doses may cause flushing and gastro-intestinal symptoms.

Nicotinyl tartrate Peripheral vasodilator acting directly on muscle in blood vessels. Used for treatment of impaired peripheral blood circulation including chilblains and Raynaud's syndrome. May cause flushing, tachycardia, shivering, gastro-intestinal symptoms, and fall in blood pressure.

Nicoumalone Anticoagulant, with actions, interactions, and adverse effects similar to **Warfarin**.

Nifedipine Antianginal/antihypertensive vasodilator. Acts by blocking influx of calcium ions into vascular smooth muscle thus reducing peripheral vascular resistance. Adverse effects include flushing, headache, and lethargy. In overdosage, causes bradycardia and hypotension, which may be treated by **Atropine**, **Dopamine**, and **Calcium gluconate**.

Nikethamide Respiratory stimulant acting directly on brain respiratory centres. Seldom useful except in respiratory depression due to severe chronic bronchitis. Not used in treatment of respiratory depression due to drug overdosage. May cause sweating, nausea, vomiting, convulsions, and depression of the nervous system.

Nimorazole Antiprotozoal used to treat certain gastro-intestinal and vaginal infections (e.g., giardiasis, trichomoniasis). Contraindicated in neurological disease. Causes nausea if alcohol taken during treatment.

Niridazole Used in treatment of infections due to the guinea worm *(Dracunculus medinensis)*. May cause gastro-intestinal symptoms, headache, and drowsiness. Rare effects include confusion, convulsions, and allergic reactions.

Nitrazepam Benzodiazepine tranquillizer/hypnotic. Depressant action on CNS. Used in treatment of insomnia. May cause dizziness, unsteadiness, and slurred speech. In overdosage, respiratory depression much less severe than with barbiturates. No antidote; supportive treatment only.

Nitrofurantoin Urinary antiseptic, producing yellow fluorescence in urine. Adverse effects include hypersensitivity reactions, nausea, vomiting, and neuropathy, haemolytic anaemia in G6PD-deficient subjects.

Nitrofurazone Antibacterial used topically for infection of the outer ear and skin wounds. Allergic reactions may occur.

Nitrophenol Has antifungal activity. Used topically for fungal infections of the skin.

Nitrous oxide Inhalational anaesthetic. Weak anaesthetic, but strong analgesic. Usually given with at least 30 percent oxygen (e.g., in dental and obstetric practice for light anaesthesia or for induction only in major surgery).

Nitrogen mustard See **Mustine hydrochloride**.

Nomifensine Antidepressant, with actions, uses, and adverse effects similar to **Imipramine**. Recently withdrawn due to increasing reports of adverse effects, including haemolytic anaemia.

Nonoxynol Nonionic surfactant used as spermicidal cream.

Nonylic acid Rubefacient used topically for musculo-skeletal pain.

Noradrenaline Sympathomimetic amine, predominantly alpha-adrenoceptor agonist. Produces general vasoconstriction with rise of blood pressure. Toxicity includes hypertension, cerebral haemorrhage, and pulmonary oedema.

Norethandrolone Sex hormone with actions similar to **Testosterone**, but anabolic effects greater than androgenic effects. Active by mouth or by injection. Used to treat debilitating conditions and carcinoma of the breast. Used with caution if liver function is impaired.

Norethisterone Sex hormone, with actions and adverse effects of **Progesterone**. Used for contraception and treatment of uterine bleeding.

Norethynodrel Sex hormone, with actions and adverse effects similar to **Progesterone**. Used for contraception and treatment of uterine bleeding.

Norgestrel Sex hormone, with actions and adverse effects similar to **Progesterone**. Used for oral contraception.

Nortriptyline Antidepressant, with actions, uses, and adverse effects similar to **Imipramine**.

Noscapine Cough suppressant, with actions and adverse effects similar to **Pholcodine**.

Novobiocin Antibiotic used for infections by **Penicillin**-resistant staphylococci. Adverse effects include hypersensitivity reactions with urticarial rashes and kernicterus in the neonate.

Noxythioline Anti-infective with antibacterial and antifungal activity. Used topically for prevention or treatment of infections in bladder or other body cavities (e.g., after bladder operations).

Nystatin Antibiotic used in treatment of *Candida* infections of skin and mucous membranes, particularly mouth, alimentary tract, and vagina.

O

Octoxynol Nonionic surfactant. Used as spermicidal cream.

Oestradiol Naturally occurring sex hormone (**Oestrogen**). Controls development and function of female sex organs, working in conjunction with **Progesterone**. Could be used for menstrual disorders, oestrogen deficiency, oral contraception, and suppression of certain neoplastic disease, but mainly superseded by related compounds. May cause withdrawal bleeding, breast development in the male, salt and water retention, nausea and vomiting, stimulation of tumours, and arterial and venous thrombosis. Use avoided in patients with known risks of these effects.

Oestriol Sex hormone (**Oestrogen**) similar to **Oestradiol**, but more active by mouth. Used mainly for menopausal disorders.

Oestrogen Sex hormone: see **Oestradiol**, **Oestriol** and **Oestrone**.

Oestrone Sex hormone (**Oestrogen**) similar to **Oestradiol**. Used mainly for menopausal disorders.

Oleandomycin Antibiotic, with similar actions and adverse effects to **Erythromycin**.

Opium tincture (c) Mixture of poppy alkaloids: see **Morphine**.

Orciprenaline Beta-adrenoceptor agonist used in bronchial asthma. Adverse effects include tachycardia, arrhythmias, and tremor.

Orphenadrine Parasympatholytic/antihistamine. Used as antispasmodic in treatment of parkinsonism. Actions, adverse effects, etc. as for **Benzhexol**.

Ouabain Plant derivative with effects on the heart similar to those of **Digoxin**, but only reliably active when given by injection when the onset of action is more rapid than for digoxin.

Oxamniquine Anti-infective for treatment of schistosomiasis due to *S. mansoni*. Adverse effects include transient fever and dizziness.

Oxatomide Antihistamine that blocks histamine H_1 receptors and release of allergic mediators from mast cells. Used in treatment of allergies (e.g., hay fever, urticaria) but not asthma. Adverse effects similar to **Promethazine** (i.e. drowsiness, potentiation of alcohol). In high doses, causes reversible weight gain.

Oxazepam Benzodiazepine anxiolytic similar to **Diazepam**.

Ox bile extract Recommended for treatment of biliary deficiency. Probably of little use, except that it increases bowel activity and helps to relieve constipation.

Oxedrine Sympathomimetic with mainly alpha-adrenergic effects. Adverse effects similar to **Noradrenaline**, but weaker and longer-acting. Recommended for treatment of hypotension.

Oxethazaine Surface-active local anaesthetic. Added to some antacid mixtures with intention of adding an analgesic effect. Actions and adverse effects similar to **Lignocaine**.

Oxolinic acid Urinary antiseptic for treatment of urine infections. May cause gastro-intestinal symptoms and CNS stimulation. Contraindicated in epilepsy.

Oxpentifylline See **Oxypentifylline**.

Oxprenolol Beta-adrenoceptor blocking drug with partial agonist activity (intrinsic sympathomimetic activity). Uses, side effects, etc. as for **Propranolol**.

Oxybuprocaine Local anaesthetic for topical use. Similar to **Amethocaine**, but less likely to cause irritation.

Oxymetazoline Sympathomimetic with marked alpha-adrenergic effects. Used topically on nasal mucosa as treatment for nasal congestion. Actions and adverse effects similar to **Naphazoline**.

Oxymetholone Sex hormone, with similar actions, uses, and adverse effects to **Testosterone**.

Oxypentifylline Vasodilator used in treatment of peripheral vascular disease (e.g., intermittent claudication, Raynaud's syndrome). May reduce blood pressure, lower blood glucose, or cause gastro-intestinal symptoms. May cause nausea, dizziness, flushing, and hypotension. Caution needed if given with antihypertensives or insulin as it may increase their effects.

Oxypertine Tranquillizer used in treatment of schizophrenia, other psychoses, and anxiety neuroses. May cause drowsiness (high doses) or hyperactivity (low doses). Gastro-intestinal disturbances, hypotension, and involuntary movements less frequent than with the phenothiazines. Coma with respiratory depression in overdosage. No antidote; supportive treatment only.

Oxyphenbutazone Anti-inflammatory/analgesic essentially similar to **Phenylbutazone** of which it is a metabolite. Now discontinued orally because of high incidence of adverse reactions. Still used topically in eye.

Oxyphenisatin Laxative used in preparative enemas before radiology, endoscopy, or surgery.

Oxyquinoline Has antibacterial, antifungal, deodorant, and keratolytic properties. Used topically on skin or in vagina for minor infections and acne. Sensitivity rashes may occur.

Oxytetracycline Bacteriostatic antibiotic, with actions, adverse effects, and interactions similar to **Tetracycline**.

Oxytocin Hormone from the posterior pituitary gland. Causes contraction of uterus. Used for induction of labour. May cause fluid retention and uterine rupture with danger to foetus. Contraindicated in toxaemia of pregnancy, placental abnormalities, or foetal distress.

P

Pancreatic enzymes Extracts of animal pancreas. Used to aid digestion of starch, fats, and protein when there is pancreatic deficiency. May cause sore mouth and sensitivity reactions with sneezing, watery eyes or skin rashes.

Pancreatin See **Pancreatic enzymes**.

Pancuronium Muscle relaxant with actions and uses similar to **Tubocurarine**.

Panthenol See **Pantothenic acid**.

Panthesine (Leucinocaine) Local anaesthetic, with actions similar to **Lignocaine**. Used as an injection in combination with protoveratrines where its hypotensive effects are said to help in the treatment of severe hypertension. See **Veratrum**.

Pantothenic acid Considered a vitamin, but no proven deficiency disease in man. No accepted therapeutic role, but included in some vitamin mixtures.

Papaveretum (c) Mixture of poppy derivatives; 50 percent is **Morphine**, to which it is similar in all respects.

Papaverine Muscle relaxant, with action on involuntary muscle. Used in bronchodilator aerosol mixtures and as relaxant in mixtures for gastrointestinal spasm. Low toxicity except intravenously when it may cause cardiac arrhythmias.

para-**Aminobenzoic acid** Nutrient. Essential metabolite for certain bacteria. Sometimes included in vitamin mixtures but there is no evidence of a deficiency disease in man. Large doses may cause nausea, skin rashes, and hypoglycaemia.

para-**Aminosalicylic acid** (PAS) Synthetic anti-tuberculous agent, usually given as the sodium salt. Adverse effects include hypersensitivity reactions, nausea, vomiting, goitre, hypothyroidism, and hepatitis.

Paracetamol (Acetaminophen–USA) Analgesic/antipyretic. Inhibits synthesis of prostaglandins in the brain but, unlike **Acetylsalicylic acid**, does not have this action in the periphery and therefore has no anti-inflammatory effect. Relieves mild pain but not inflammation. Overdosage may cause potentially fatal liver damage. **Cysteamine** and **Methionine** may be of value as antidotes.

Paradichlorobenzene Insecticide included in some ear drops. May irritate the skin. Inhalation or ingestion may cause drowsiness.

Paraldehyde Anticonvulsant/hypnotic/sedative. Used in status epilepticus or disturbed patients. Administered by intramuscular injection. Dissolves plastic syringes: glass must be used. Irritant at injection site. Exhaled in breath producing unpleasant odour.

Parathyroid hormone Extract from parathyroid glands. Increases plasma calcium by mobilizing calcium from bone, reducing urine calcium excretion, and increasing its absorption from the gastro-intestinal tract. Active only by injection. Used to treat low plasma calcium (tetany). May cause abnormally high plasma calcium with weakness, lethargy, and coma.

Pargyline Monoamine oxidase inhibitor. Reduces blood pressure by unknown mechanism. Antihypertensive. Shares adverse interactions of **Phenelzine** and may produce fluid retention.

PAS See *para*-**Aminosalicylic acid**.

Pectin Emulsifying agent, used in preparation of pharmaceutical and cosmetic products.

Pemoline CNS stimulant with action intermediate between **Caffeine** and **Amphetamine**. Used as treatment for lethargy. May cause insomnia, anxiety, and rapid heart rate.

Penamecillin Similar to **Phenoxymethylpenicillin**.

Penbutolol Non-selective beta-adrenoceptor blocking drug, with actions, uses, and adverse effects similar to **Propranolol**. Long half-life permits once daily dosage.

Penicillamine Chelating agent. Binds certain toxic metals (e.g., copper) and increases their excretion. Used in treatment of metal poisoning and rheumatoid arthritis (where its mechanism of action is uncertain). May cause headache, fever, loss of taste, gastro-intestinal symptoms, kidney damage, and bone marrow depression.

Penicillins Group of bactericidal antibiotics that act by inhibiting bacterial cell wall synthesis. Hypersensitivity cross-reactions occur to all.

Penicillin V See **Phenoxymethylpenicillin**.

Pentaerythritol tetranitrate Vasodilator with longer, but milder, action than **Glyceryl trinitrate** whose adverse effects it shares. Used to prevent angina attacks.

Pentagastrin Synthetic gastro-intestinal hormone. Stimulates secretion of gastric acid, pepsin and pancreatic enzymes. Used by injection as test of gastric and pancreatic function. May cause nausea, flushing, dizziness, and fall in blood pressure.

Pentamidine Used in treatment of leishmaniasis. Adverse effects include hypotension, nausea, and vomiting.

Pentazocine Narcotic analgesic more potent than **Codeine**, but less potent than **Morphine**. Dependence and addiction less common than with **Morphine**. Some activity as a narcotic antagonist like **Naloxone**. May cause bad dreams, hallucinations, withdrawal symptoms, also nausea, vomiting, dizziness, and drowsiness. Constipation, and rarely respiratory depression may occur after injections. **Naloxone** but not **Nalorphine** nor **Levallorphan** may be used as antagonists.

Penthienate Anticholinergic, with actions and adverse effects similar to **Atropine**. Used to relieve gastro-intestinal spasm.

Pentobarbitone (c) Barbiturate hypnotic essentially like **Amylobarbitone**.

Peppermint oil Essential oil used to relieve gastric and intestinal flatulence and colic. Adverse effects include allergic reactions to its menthol content.

Pepsin Enzyme found in normal gastric juice. Controls breakdown of proteins. May be given to improve digestion when there is deficiency of pepsin secretion.

Perhexilene Antianginal agent. Used for prevention of symptoms but not treatment of acute attack. May cause nerve damage, liver damage, dizziness, nausea, vomiting, weakness, flushing, and skin rashes.

Pericyazine Tranquillizer, with actions, uses, and adverse effects similar tc **Chlorpromazine**.

Perphenazine Phenothiazine tranquillizer similar to **Chlorpromazine** used in treatment of psychotic disorders, agitation, and confusion. Not recommended for children.

Pethidine (c) Synthetic narcotic analgesic essentially similar to **Morphine**. Used for relief of severe pain. May produce nausea, vomiting, dry mouth, euphoria, sedation, and respiratory depression. Coma with danger of death on overdosage. **Naxolone** is a specific antagonist. Long-term use associated with tolerance, physical dependence, and ('addiction') abuse.

PGI_2 See **Epoprostenol**.

Phenacetin Analgesic/antipyretic, but not anti-inflammatory. Converted by the liver to **Paracetamol** which is the main active form. Available only in combined analgesic preparations. Does not cause gastric irritation but may cause haemolytic anaemia and methaemoglobinaemia. Has been associated with kidney damage (analgesic nephropathy) and is now seldom used in UK.

Phenazocine (c) Narcotic analgesic similar to **Morphine**, but causes less sedation, vomiting, and hypotension. More likely to depress respiration than morphine.

Phenazone Analgesic/antipyretic. Local anaesthetic action when applied topically. Not much used but found in some analgesic mixtures and in ear drops. May cause skin rashes and bone marrow suppression. Overdose may result in nausea, coma, and convulsions. The rate of metabolism (half-life) of single doses is sometimes used as a measure of drug metabolism by the liver.

Phenazopyridine Analgesic recommended for relief of pain and irritation in the urinary tract (e.g., cystitis). Causes orange or red coloration of urine. May cause headache, dizziness, and blood disorders. Contraindicated in renal or liver failure.

Phenbenicillin As for **Phenoxymethylpenicillin**.

Phencyclidine Drug of abuse commonly known as 'Angel Dust'. Originally used as an aid to anaesthesia, but found to cause pronounced psychotic effects which are usually unpleasant.

Phenelzine Antidepressant; inhibits monoamine oxidase thus increasing tissue concentrations of **Noradrenaline**, **Dopamine**, and 5-hydroxytryptamine. Adverse effects include hepatitis, interactions with tyramine-containing foods, and indirect sympathomimetic amines producing hypertensive crises, and with narcotics to produce profound CNS depression. Hypertensive crisis treated with alpha-adrenoceptor blocker (e.g., **Phentolamine**).

Phenethicillin Similar to **Phenoxymethylpenicillin**.

Phenindamine Antihistamine, with actions and uses similar to **Promethazine**. Unlike most antihistamines, it causes stimulant side effects and may be used when sedation is a problem. May cause insomnia, convulsions, dry mouth, and gastro-intestinal disturbances.

Phenindione Anticoagulant, with actions and interactions similar to **Warfarin**. Adverse effects include allergic reactions, jaundice, and steatorrhoea.

Pheniramine Antihistamine, with actions, uses, and adverse effects similar to **Promethazine**.

Phenmetrazine (c) Anorectic/sympathomimetic amine, widely abused, with actions and adverse effects of **Amphetamine**.

Phenobarbitone (c) (Phenobarbital–USA) Long-acting barbiturate anticonvulsant. Depresses epileptic discharges in the brain. Used orally as preventive treatment in epileptics and occasionally by injection to control a severe fit. Danger of sedation and impairment of learning capacity. Induces its own metabolism by the liver. Given only with caution in liver disease. Danger of drug interaction. Coma with respiratory depression in overdose. No antidote. Treatment is supportive, sometimes plus forced alkaline diuresis or haemodialysis to promote excretion of the drug.

Phenol Disinfectant in dilute solution; in strong solutions it denatures cell proteins and damages sensory nerves. Used include injection for the sclerosis of haemorrhoids and alleviation of intractable pain by localized effects in the nerves involved.

Phenolphthalein Purgative that acts by direct stimulation of colonic muscle. Action prolonged by absorption of drug from the gut and recirculation in bile. Produces pink urine and faeces (red if alkaline). May cause skin rashes in sensitive individuals.

Phenoperidine (c) Narcotic analgesic, with actions and adverse effects similar to **Morphine**. Used with **Droperidol** to produce neuroleptanalgesia–a state of consciousness but calmness and indifference–allowing the patient to cooperate with the surgeon.

Phenoxybenzamine Alkylating agent with alpha-adrenoceptor blocking and antihistamine effects. Used in phaeochromocytoma. Side effects include sedation, nausea, and vomiting.

Phenoxybenzylpenicillin (Phenbenicillin) As for **Phenoxymethylpenicillin**.

Phenoxyethylpenicillin (Phenethicillin) As for **Phenoxymethylpenicillin**.

Phenoxymethylpenicillin (Penicillin V) Acid-resistant **Penicillin** used orally. Shares actions and adverse effects of **Benzylpenicillin**.

Phenoxypropanol Preservative/anti-infective for skin preparations.

Phenoxypropylpenicillin (Propicillin) As for **Phenoxymethylpenicillin**.

Phensuximide Anticonvulsant essentially similar to **Ethosuximide**.

Phentermine (c) Anorectic/Sympathomimetic amine. Actions and adverse effects similar to **Diethylpropion**.

Phentolamine Alpha-adrenoceptor blocking drug with partial agonist and smooth muscle relaxant activity. Used in phaeochromocytoma. Side effects include tachycardia and nasal stuffiness.

Phenylbutazone Anti-inflammotory/analgesic used in treatment of inflammotory joint disorders. Adverse effects include nausea, vomiting, skin rashes, peptic ulceration, sodium retention, and hypotension. Occasionally causes bone marrow depression with thrombocytopaenia, agranulocytosis, and aplastic anaemia. May enhance action of oral anticoagulants (e.g., **Warfarin**). Owing to high incidence of adverse effects, its use has been restricted to one condition only, ankylosing spondylitis.

Phenylephrine Sympathomimetic amine, with actions, uses, and toxicity of **Noradrenaline**. Also used as mydriatic and nasal decongestant.

Phenylpropanolamine Sympathomimetic, with actions, uses, and adverse effects similar to **Ephedrine**.

Phenyltoloxamine Antihistamine, with actions, uses, and adverse effects similar to **Promethazine**.

Phenytoin Anticonvulsant. Suppresses epileptic discharge in the brain. Used orally to prevent convulsions and by injection to control convulsions or to suppress irregular heart rhythms. Long-term use may cause gum hypertrophy, acne, hirsutism, folate deficiency, anaemia, osteomalacia, and liver enzyme induction with danger of drug interactions. In mild overdosage, causes ataxia, dysarthria, and nystagmus. Coma and respiratory depression in severe cases. No antidote; supportive therapy only.

Pholcodine Narcotic derivative related to **Codeine** but with little analgesic activity. Used only for cough suppression. May cause constipation. Similar to **Codeine** in overdosage.

Phosphoric acid In dilute form acts as a stimulant to gastric secretion.

Phosphorylcolamine Synthetic amino acid with high phosphorus content. Said to promote improved metabolism. Used as a 'tonic' in debilitated patients.

Phthalylsulphathiazole Sulphonamide antibacterial with actions, etc. of **Sulphadimidine** Poorly absorbed. Used mainly for gut infections and sterilization.

Physostigmine (Eserine) Anticholinesterase, allowing accumulation of

Acetylcholine. Actions those of **Acetylcholine**. Effects of overdose antagonized by **Atropine**.

Phytomenadione See **Vitamin K**.

Pilocarpine Parasympathomimetic drug, with actions of **Acetylcholine**.

Pimozide Tranquillizer, with uses, adverse effects, etc. similar to **Chlorpromazine**.

Pindolol Beta-adrenoceptor blocking drug with partial agonist activity (intrinsic sympathomimetic activity). Uses, side effects, etc. as for **Propranolol**.

Pipenzolate Anticholinergic, with actions and adverse effects similar to **Atropine**. Used to reduce gastric acid secretion and intestinal spasm.

Piperacillin Broad-spectrum, injectable **Penicillin** similar to **Carbenicillin**, particularly effective against gram-negative organisms including *Pseudomonas, Proteus*, anaerobes. Used in severe, life-threatening infections. Adverse effects similar to **Benzylpenicillin**. Dosage reduction needed in renal failure.

Piperazine Used in treatment of threadworms and roundworms. Adverse effects include dizziness and ataxia.

Piperidolate Anticholinergic, with actions and adverse effects similar to **Atropine**. Relatively weak. Used to decrease gastro-intestinal motility and spasm.

Pipothiazine Phenothiazine tranquillizer, with indications, actions, and adverse effects similar to **Fluphenazine**.

Pirbuterol Bronchoselective beta-adrenoceptor agonist, with actions, uses, and adverse effects similar to **Salbutamol**.

Pirenzepine Anticholinergic with selective effects on gastric mucosa. Reduces gastric acid secretion while causing less of the adverse effects normally associated with such compounds (see **Atropine**). May cause dry mouth and blurred vision.

Piretanide Diuretic, with actions, uses, and adverse effects similar to **Frusemide**.

Piroxicam Non-steroid anti-inflammatory/analgesic with long duration of action needing only once daily dosage. Actions and uses similar to **Ibuprofen**. Adverse effects include gastro-intestinal intolerance and oedema.

Pituitary gland extract Extract of animal pituitary tissue used for its anti-diuretic activity. See **Vasopressin**.

Pivampicillin Prodrug antibiotic. Readily absorbed from gastro-intestinal tract and rapidly metabolized to the active drug **Ampicillin**, whose actions, uses, and adverse effects it shares.

Pivmecillinam Prodrug antibiotic. Readily absorbed from gastro-intestinal tract and rapidly metabolized to the active drug **Mecillinam**, whose actions, uses, and adverse effects it shares.

Pizotifen For prevention of migraine. Has antiserotonin and antihistamine properties. May cause drowsiness, weight gain, dizziness, and nausea.

Podophyllin Plant extract resin, with antimitotic and purgative actions. Used topically to treat warts and by mouth as an irritant purgative (mainly succeeded by less irritant compounds.

Podophyllum Purgative. Pronounced irritant effect on the bowel or skin. Because of its violent effects has been replaced by milder drugs. Still used as a paint for warts where it prevents growth.

Poldine Parasympatholytic, with actions, etc. similar to **Atropine**. Used to reduce gastric acid secretion in treatment of peptic ulceration.

Poloxalene Purgative. Lowers surface tension of intestinal fluids and softens faeces.

Poloxamer '188' See **Poloxalene**.

Polyethylene glycol Used as a solvent and/or moisturizing agent in topical preparations.

Polymyxin B Antibiotic active against gram-negative bacteria. Not absorbed when taken by mouth but effective topically (e.g., within gut or on skin or eyes). May also be given by intramuscular injection. Rarely causes skin sensitivity but injections may be painful and associated with neurological symptoms.

Polynoxylin Antiseptic, with wide antibacterial and antifungal actions. Used topically for skin, throat, and external ear infections.

Polyoestradiol Sex hormone. Used in treatment of carcinoma of the prostate. Adverse effects similar to **Ethinyloestradiol**.

Polysaccharide–iron complex Haematinic, with actions, uses, and adverse effects similar to **Ferrous sulphate**.

Polysorbate 60 Emulsifying agent. Aids water-in-oil mixtures and solubilizing of fat-soluble substances.

Polythiazide Thiazide diuretic similar to **Bendrofluazide**.

Polyvinyl alcohol A synthetic resin with strong hydrophilic properties used in eye drops to lubricate dry eyes and in jelly skin preparations which dry rapidly to form a soluble plastic film.

Posterior pituitary extract Mixed hormonal extract, with actions of **Oxytocin** and **Vasopressin** whose toxic effects it also shares. Used by injection or nasal absorption to treat diabetes insipidus.

Potassium aluminium sulphate See **Alum**.

Potassium bicarbonate Antacid. Has been used as gastric antacid as **Sodium bicarbonate**, but unsuitable for intravenous use.

Potassium canrenoate Potassium-sparing diuretic, related to, and with similar actions, uses, and adverse effects to **Spironolactone**.

Potassium chloride Potassium supplement. Used when there is a danger of hypokalaemia (e.g., treatment with potassium-losing diuretics) and fluid overload in liver failure. Oral potassium chloride itself causes nausea and gastric irritation. Usually administered as slow-release preparation or in an effervescent solution of bicarbonate and trimethylglycine. May be given by slow intravenous infusion. Danger of hyperkalaemia in renal failure. Treated by haemodialysis and ion exchange resins.

Potassium citrate Renders urine less acid. Used to reduce bladder inflammation. May produce adverse effects similar to **Potassium chloride**.

Potassium guaiacolsulphonate Expectorant included in certain cough mixtures.

Potassium *para*-aminobenzoate Nutrient. See ***para*-Aminobenzoic acid.** Has been used to treat skin disorders where there is excessive fibrosis (e.g., scleroderma).

Potassium perchlorate Treatment for overactive thyroid gland. Reduces formation of thyroid hormone by interfering with uptake of iodine into the gland. May cause nausea, vomiting, rashes, kidney damage, and bone marrow suppression.

Povidone-iodine Antiseptic. Liberates inorganic iodine slowly onto the skin or mucous membranes. Used pre-operatively and in treatment of wounds.

Practolol Cardioselective beta-adrenoceptor blocking drug. Withdrawn because of adverse effects on eye, ear, and peritoneum.

Pralidoxime (P2S) Cholinesterase reactivator used in treatment of organophosphorus cholinesterase poisoning.

Pramoxine Surface-active local anaesthetic, with actions and adverse effects similar to **Lignocaine**. Used topically on skin or mucous membranes.

Prazepam Benzodiazepine, with actions and toxic effects similar to **Diazepam**. Used to treat anxiety states and muscle spasms.

Praziquantel Anti-infective for treatment of schistosomiasis. Active against *S. haematobium* and *S. japonicum*. Effective both in urinary tract and hepatic infections. Adverse effects, usually transient, include nausea, epigastric pain, dizziness, and drowsiness.

Prazosin Vasodilator/antihypertensive. Adverse effects include tachycardia and headache. Excessive fall in blood pressure may occur early in treatment.

Prednisolone Synthetic **Corticosteroid**, with actions, etc. as for **Prednisone**.

Prednisone Synthetic **Corticosteroid**, with similar actions, etc. to **Cortisone**, but has greater anti-inflammatory activity with less salt and water retention.

Prenalterol Synthetic beta-adrenoceptor agonist which increases the force of cardiac contraction with only minor increases in heart rate and little, if any, peripheral vascular actions. Used in intractable heart failure. May be useful as antidote in overdosage of beta-adrenoceptor antagonists.

Prenylamine Vasodilator used to prevent angina attacks. May cause gastro-intestinal symptoms, flushing, skin rashes, and hypotension. Contra-indicated in cardiac or liver failure.

Prilocaine Local anaesthetic similar to **Lignocaine**, but less toxic. Used in dentistry.

Primaquine Antimalarial agent. Adverse effects include nausea, methaemoglobinaemia, and haemolytic anaemia.

Primidone Anticonvulsant. Similar to barbiturates; partly metabolized by liver to **Phenobarbitone**. Suppresses epileptic discharges in the brain. Used orally to prevent convulsions. Additive effect with **Phenobarbitone** to which it is otherwise essentially similar.

Probenecid For prevention of gout. Increases urine excretion of uric acid and thus reduces its levels in the body. May cause nausea, vomiting, and skin rashes. Reduces excretion of **Penicillin**.

Probucol Reduces elevated concentrations of serum cholesterol with lesser effect on triglycerides. Used in hypercholesterolaemia.

Procainamide Antidysrhythmic/local anaesthetic similar to **Procaine** but longer-acting and with less CNS stimulation. Used to treat cardiac dysrhythmias, but contraindicated in heart block. May cause dose-related hypotension, mental depression, and hallucinations. Hypersensitivity may cause arthritis and rash (systemic lupus erythematosus-like syndrome).

Procaine Local anaesthetic. Stabilizes nerve cell membranes to prevent impulse transmission. Used by injection for anaesthesia in minor operations. Poor activity if applied topically. Short action (due to rapid removal in the blood) may be prolonged by combination with a vasoconstrictor (e.g., **Adrenaline**). May cause CNS stimulation with euphoria and convulsions. Metabolite of procaine interferes with antimicrobial activity of sulphonamides (e.g., **Sulphadimidine**). Preparations containing adrenaline are contraindicated in heart disease, hyperthyroidism, or treatment with tricyclic antidepressants (e.g., **Amitriptyline**) where it may cause cardiac dysrhythmias.

Procaine penicillin Long-acting form of **Benzylpenicillin**, with similar actions and adverse effects.

Procarbazine Cytotoxic drug used in neoplastic disease. Adverse effects include nausea, vomiting, diarrhoea, stomatitis, alopecia, neurotoxicity, and bone marrow depression.

Prochlorperazine Phenothiazine similar to **Chlorpromazine**, but less sedative and more potent anti-emetic actions. Used mainly as an anti-emetic. More likely than **Chlorpromazine** to cause extrapyramidal side effects. May be given orally, by injection, or as suppository.

Procyclidine Parasympatholytic used in treatment of parkinsonism. Actions, etc. similar to **Benzhexol**.

Progesterone Sex hormone acts on the uterus (in sequence with **Oestrogen**) to prepare the endometrium to receive the fertilized ovum. Has been used in treatment of uterine bleeding, for contraception, for breast and uterine tumours, and for threatened abortion. Has to be injected and therefore largely replaced by newer progestational agents which are active by mouth. May cause acne, weight gain, enlargements of the breasts, gastrointestinal symptoms, and jaundice.

Proguanil Antimalarial agent. Adverse effects include vomiting and renal irritation.

Prolintane CNS stimulant claimed to have effect intermediate between **Caffeine** and **Amphetamine**. Used to treat lethargy. May cause nausea, rapid heart rate, and insomnia.

Promazine Phenothiazine/antihistamine similar to **Chlorpromazine**.

Promethazine Phenothiazine/antihistamine with actions similar to **Chlorpromazine**. Used as an anti-emetic and in treatment of allergic reactions, but has little antipsychotic effects. Marked sedative effects make it useful as a hypnotic in children and in pre-operative medication. Adverse effects and overdosage effects similar to **Chlorpromazine**.

Propamidine Antiseptic, with antibacterial and antifungal actions. Used topically for infections of skin and conjunctiva. Treatment should not be prolonged more than one week or tissue damage may occur.

Propantheline Parasympatholytic, with peripheral and toxic effects similar to **Atropine**. Used to reduce gastric acid secretion in peptic ulceration and as an antispasmodic for gastro-intestinal and urinary complaints. Contraindications and overdosage effects as for **Atropine**.

Propicillin Essentially similar to **Phenoxymethylpenicillin**.

Propranolol Beta-adrenoceptor antagonist used in angina, hypertension, arrhythmias, hyperthyroidism, migraine and anxiety. May cause bronchoconstriction, cardiac failure, and cold extremities and sleep disturbances.

Propylene glycol Solvent used in extract of some crude drugs and as a vehicle for some injections and topical applications. May cause local irritation but less toxic than other glycols owing to rapid breakdown and excretion.

Propylhexedrine Sympathomimetic used as inhalation for treatment of nasal congestion. Actions and adverse effects similar to **Naphazoline**.

Propylthiouracil Depresses formation of thyroid hormone. Used in treatment of hyperthyroidism. Adverse effects include allergic rashes, headache, nausea, diarrhoea, and blood dyscrasias, including tendency to bleeding.

Prostacyclin See **Epoprostenol**.

Protamine sulphate Specific antidote to anticoagulant effect of **Heparin**. Derived from fish protein. Adverse effects include hypotension and dyspnoea.

Prothionamide Anti-tuberculous agent, with actions and uses similar to **Ethionamide**. May be better tolerated.

Protirelin Also known as thyrotrophin-releasing-hormone (TRH). Used intravenously as a diagnostic agent in difficult cases of hypothyroidism where it causes a rapid rise of plasma **thyrotrophin** (TSH) in normal cases.

Protriptyline Antidepressant, with similar action and adverse effects to **Imipramine** but has central stimulating effects. Used to treat depression associated with withdrawal and lack of energy. May aggravate anxiety and insomnia.

Proxymetacaine Surface-active, local anaesthetic with actions and adverse effects similar to **Lignocaine**. Used in ophthalmology.

Proxyphylline Bronchodilator, with actions and uses similar to **Aminophylline**. Said to cause fewer gastro-intestinal symptoms.

Pseudoephedrine Sympathomimetic, with actions, uses, and adverse effects similar to **Ephedrine**. Used mainly as decongestant. Said to have less effect on increasing blood pressure.

Psyllium Purgative. Increases faecal bulk by same mechanism as **Methylcellulose**.

Pyrantel Antiworm treatment. Acts by paralyzing mature and immature forms, thus allowing their excretion. Little absorbed from the gut so that its activity is concentrated where needed at the site of the infection. Used as a single dose for threadworm, hookworm, roundworm, whipworm and trichostrongyliasis. May cause gastro-intestinal disturbances, headache, dizziness, drowsiness, insomnia, and rashes.

Pyrazinamide Anti-tuberculous drug. High incidence of adverse effects, particularly liver toxicity.

Pyridostigmine Anticholinesterase, with actions similar to **Physostigmine**.

Pyridoxine (Vitamin B_6) Vitamin used in treatment of specific deficiency and other anaemias and in **Isoniazid**-induced neuropathy. Recommended also for depression due to the oral contraceptive but true pyridoxine deficiency is not universal in such cases.

Pyrimethamine Antimalarial agent. Adverse effects include skin rashes and folate-deficient anaemia.

Q

Quinalbarbitone (c) Barbiturate hypnotic usually prescribed in combined preparation with **Amylobarbitone**. No major differences from **Amylobarbitone**.

Quinestradol Sex hormone (**Oestrogen**) similar to **Oestradiol**. Claimed to have greater effect on the vagina than on the uterus or breast. Used for postmenopausal vaginitis.

Quinestrol Sex hormone (**Oestrogen**) similar to **Oestradiol**. Used for suppression of lactation and menopausal disorders.

Quinidine Antidysrhythmic agent, with local anaesthetic activity. Depresses myocardial contractility and impulse conduction. Reduces cardiac output. Used to prevent recurrent dysrhythmias or to convert established dysrythmias back to normal sinus rhythm. Dose-dependent effects include vertigo, tinnitus, deafness, blurred vision, confusion, gastrointestinal symptoms, cardiac arrhythmias, and cardiac arrest. Rashes and bruising are dose-independent. Contraindicated when dysrhythmia is due to **Digoxin** or when there is heart block.

Quinine Antimalarial agent. Used to reduce skeletal muscle spasms. Adverse effects include vomiting, psychosis, visual and auditory disturbances, haemolytic anaemia, and thrombocytopenia. Toxic doses may cause abortion.

R

Ranitidine Selectively blocks histamine receptors mediating gastric acid secretions. Uses and adverse effects similar to **Cimetidine**, but may cause less CNS effects or breast enlargement in males.

Rauwolfia Indian shrub. See **Reserpine** for main derivative.

Razoxane Antimitotic used in treatment of certain bone and soft-tissue tumours together with radiotherapy. May cause gastro-intestinal disturbance, bone marrow suppression, and hair loss.

Reproterol Beta-adrenoceptor agonist, with actions, uses, and adverse effects as for **Salbutamol**.

Reserpine Rauwolfia derivative. Reduces sympathetic tone by **Noradrenaline** depletion. Depletes brain **Noradrenaline**, **Dopamine**, and 5-hydroxytryptamine. Used in hypertension and as antipsychotic. Adverse effects include depression, parkinsonism, nasal stuffiness, fluid retention, and impotence.

Resorcinol Dermatological treatment. Reduces itching and helps remove scaly skin. Used topically in treatment of acne and dandruff. Also as ear drops where used for antiseptic effects. If absorbed over long term, may cause suppression of thyroid gland. If ingested, is corrosive and may cause kidney damage, coma, and convulsions.

Retinol See **Vitamin A**.

Riboflavine (Vitamin B_2) Vitamin. Deficiency leads to mucosal ulceration and angular stomatitis.

Ricinoleic acid Acid that forms stable soaps with alkalis. Used in contraceptive creams and jellies.

Rifampicin Bactericidal antibiotic, used in tuberculosis. Adverse effects include liver toxicity and influenza-like symptoms. Induces liver enzymes, so reducing effectiveness of oral contraceptives and corticosteroids.

Rimiterol Beta-adrenoceptor agonist. Actions, uses, and adverse effects as for **Salbutamol**.

Ritodrine Beta-adrenoceptor agonist. Actions, uses, and adverse effects as for **Isoxsuprine**.

Rose bengal Staining agent. Used for detection of damage to the cornea.

Rubella vaccine Live attenuated rubella virus for immunization against rubella (German measles). Used routinely in girls before puberty. May be used in non-pregnant women of child-bearing age. Adverse effects include rash, fever, enlarged lymph glands, joint pains. Must not be given to pregnant women or those receiving drugs to suppress the immune response.

Rubidomycin See **Daunorubicin**.

S

Salbutamol Bronchoselective beta-adrenoceptor agonist used in bronchial asthma by inhalation, intravenous infusion or orally. Used also by intravenous infusion or orally to inhibit premature labour. Adverse effects include tachycardia, arrhythmias, tremors, and muscle cramps.

Salcatonin Hormone derived from salmon, or by synthesis, with actions, uses, and adverse effects similar to **Calcitonin**.

Salicylamide Analgesic/antipyretic, with actions and adverse effects similar to **Acetylsalicylic acid** but less effective and used only infrequently. In overdosage, does not cause acidosis but depression of respiration and loss of consciousness.

Salicylic acid Anti-inflammatory/analgesic; an active metabolite of **Acetylsalicylic acid** whose adverse effects it shares. Not used systemically as it causes marked gastric irritation. Topically on skin it acts as a keratolytic and has bacteriostatic and antifungal properties. Used to treat warts, skin ulcers, psoriasis, and other skin conditions.

Salsalate Anti-inflammatory/analgesic. After absorption is broken down to **Salicylic acid**. Uses and adverse effects similar to **Acetylsalicylic acid**.

Selegiline Selective monoamine oxidase inhibitor, which prevents breakdown of **Dopamine** in the brain and so increases and prolongs the action of **Levodopa**. Used in conjunction with **Levodopa** in the treatment of Parkinson's disease. Adverse effects include hypotension, nausea, vomiting, confusion, agitation, and involuntary movements.

Selenium sulphide Reduces formation of dandruff and other forms of eczema of the scalp. Used as a shampoo. Highly toxic if ingested causing anorexia, garlic breath, vomiting, anaemia, and liver damage.

Senna Plant extract purgative, with actions, adverse effects, etc. as for **Cascara**.

Sennosides A and B Active principles of **Senna**.

Silver nitrate Disinfectant/cleansing agent, used in wet dressings or baths for suppurating lesions. Must only be used short-term. The lotion should not be used if a precipitate is present.

Silver protein Has mild antibacterial properties. Used in eye drops or nasal sprays for treatment of minor infections.

Silver sulphadiazine Sulphonamide derivative, with actions similar to **Sulphadimidine**. Used topically in treatment of burns to prevent infection.

Simethicone Silicone/silica mixture used for water-repellent and anti-foaming properties. Included in barrier creams and in oral treatments for flatulence.

Soap spirit Soft soap in alcohol used in some dermatological preparations for its cleaning and descaling actions.

Sodium acid citrate Anticoagulant. Now preferred to **Sodium citrate**.

Sodium acid phosphate Saline purgative, with actions and uses similar to **Sodium phosphate**.

Sodium alkyl sulphoacetate Wetting agent/laxative. Used mainly as an enema for treatment of persistent constipation and pre-operative bowel evacuation.

Sodium antimonylgluconate (Triostam) Used in schistosomiasis. Adverse effects include anorexia, nausea, vomiting, diarrhoea, muscle and joint pains, and cardiotoxicity.

Sodium aurothiomalate Used in rheumatic diseases, notably severe rheumatoid arthritis where it is capable of halting the disease process. Given intramuscularly in weekly doses, it takes up to four to six months to achieve maximum effect. Adverse effects include mouth ulcers, skin rashes, oedema, proteinuria, blood dyscrasias, colitis, peripheral neuritis, and pulmonary fibrosis. The high incidence of adverse effects can be reduced if use of this drug is controlled from specialist rheumatology centres.

Sodium bicarbonate Absorbable (systemic) antacid. Rapidly dissolves and neutralizes acid in stomach. Produces quick relief of dyspepsia due to peptic ulceration but is not retained in stomach and therefore has short duration of action. Absorbed from small intestine, may cause systemic alkalosis. If used in large doses, with large doses of milk may cause renal damage (i.e. 'milk–alkali syndrome'). Danger of fluid retention in patients with cardiac failure or renal disease.

Sodium calcium edetate Chelating agent. Exchanges its calcium for other metal ions in the blood. Most effective exchange is for lead and it may be used by injection or by mouth for treatment of lead poisoning. May cause nausea, diarrhoea, abdominal cramps, and pain and thrombophlebitis at site of injection. Renal damage and dermatitis have occurred with prolonged treatment. Used with caution if there is pre-existing renal disease.

Sodium cellulose phosphate Nonabsorbable powder taken by mouth in treatment of hypercalcaemia. Adsorbs calcium ions in the intestine and prevents their absorption thus reducing the dietary intake of calcium.

Sodium chloride Essential component of body fluids and tissues. Used intravenously to replace lost fluids when rapid treatment is needed or orally when replacement is less urgent (e.g., for sweat loss in tropics). Hyperosmolar solutions have been recommended as an emetic for first-aid treatment of poisoning, but saline is a poor emetic and may cause death due to hypernatraemia. This use is no longer recommended.

Sodium citrate Mild purgative used in some enemas. Was used as an anticoagulant in blood for transfusion but now superseded by **Sodium acid citrate**.

Sodium cromoglycate Preventive treatment for asthma, rhintis (hay fever), and conjunctivitis due to allergy. Also used for ulcerative colitis. Acts by blocking allergic mechanisms. Administered orally, by inhalation of powder or topically in eye. May cause bronchial irritation and spasm, and contact dermititis..

Sodium edetate Chelating agent used intravenously to reduce high blood calcium levels. Actions and adverse effects similar to **Sodium calcium edetate**. May cause excessive lowering of calcium levels.

Sodium fluoride Used for the prevention of dental caries in areas where the intake of fluoride from drinking water is low. May be given in water or fruit juice or applied to the teeth in solution or toothpaste. Adverse effects occur only in overdosage or from high environmental fluoride levels. Large overdoses may cause gastro-intestinal symptoms, paralysis and convulsions, with death from cardiac and respiratory failure. Chronic poisoning may cause increased bone density and eye damage.

Sodium hyaluronate Transparent, high-viscosity sodium salt of high-molecular-weight carbohydrate. Used in ophthalmic surgery to replace aqueous and vitreous humour.

Sodium hypochlorite Source of chlorine, which has antimicrobial action for cleansing and desloughing of skin ulcers.

Sodium iodide Expectorant. Causes increased and more watery bronchial secretion. Included in some cough mixtures. Acts also as a source of iodine (essential for production of thyroid hormone). Added to table salt to prevent endemic goitre and may be used pre-operatively to prepare hyperactive goitre for removal. Should not be given in pulmonary tuberculosis where it may reactivate the disease.

Sodium iron edetate Haematinic, with actions, uses, and adverse effects similar to **Ferrous sulphate**.

Sodium lactate Salt administered intravenously to increase the alkali reserve. Metabolized to bicarbonate. Contraindicated in liver failure, where conversion to bicarbonate is impaired.

Sodium lauryl sulphate Detergent/wetting agent. Used for cleaning properties in skin preparations and in enemas to aid softening of faeces.

Sodium lauryl sulphoacetate Similar to **Sodium lauryl sulphate**.

Sodium morrhuate Sclerosing agent used for injection treatment of varicose veins; causes obliteration of the dilated vessels. May cause allergic reactions. A test dose is recommended.

Sodium nitroprusside Potent, rapid-acting antihypertensive used by intravenous infusion for severe hypertensive crisis or for controlled hypotension during surgical procedures. Acts by direct dilatation of blood vessels. Duration brief as metabolized to cyanide and then thiocyanate. Adverse effects include sweating, nausea, vomiting, weakness, and muscle twitching. Excessive dosage may lead to 'cyanide poisoning' (i.e. tachycardia, hyperventilation, cardiac arrhythmias plus the above symptoms). **Cobalt edetate** or **sodium nitrite** plus **sodium thiosulphate** are antidotes.

Sodium perborate Mild disinfectant/deodorant used for mouth infections. Prolonged use may cause blistering and swelling in mouth.

Sodium phosphate Saline purgative. Poorly absorbed from the gastrointestinal tract. Retains water in the intestine and thus increases faecal mass.

Sodium picosulphate Saline purgative with actions and uses similar to **Magnesium sulphate**.

Sodium polystyrene sulphonate Ion exchange resin used in treatment of high plasma potassium levels where it exchanges sodium ions for potassium. May be used orally or rectally. Adverse effects include nausea, vomiting, constipation, and sodium overload which may cause cardiac failure.

Sodium pyrrolidone-carboxylate Hygroscopic salt. Used as a moisturing agent for dry skin.

Sodium ricinoleate Surface-active agent used in some toothpastes for its cleaning properties.

Sodium salicylate Analgesic/anti-inflammatory/antipyretic, with actions, uses, and adverse effects similar to **Acetylsalicylic acid**. Usually taken in solution. Danger of sodium overload in patients with cardiac failure or renal failure.

Sodium sulphate (Glauber's salts) Saline purgative. Actions and uses similar to **Magnesium sulphate**. Unpleasant taste. Danger of sodium retention with congestive heart failure in susceptible subjects.

Sodium tetradecyl sulphate Injection used for treatment of varicose veins.

Sodium valproate Anticonvulsant. May act by increasing brain levels of gamma-aminobutyric acid (GABA). Used in all forms of epilepsy. May cause gastro-intestinal symptoms, liver necrosis, and prolonged bleeding times with thrombocytopaenia. Before surgery, check for bleeding tendencies. May potentiate effects of antidepressant drugs whose dose should be reduced in combined treatment.

Soft paraffin Topical emollient and protective used on skin in 'barrier creams' and wound dressings where it aids removal of the dressing.

Somatotrophin (Growth hormone) Human growth hormone. Extracted from pituitary glands. Used to treat short stature when the epiphyses remain open. Available only from special centres.

Somatrem Synthetic hormone with actions similar to growth hormone (**Somatotrophin**). Produced by genetic engineering (DNA recombinant technology). Replaces growth hormones extracted from human pituitary glands and thus avoids the risk of viral infections from that source. Used in treatment of short stature due to growth hormone deficiency. Should not be used in patients with diabetes mellitus or those whose bone epiphyses have closed.

Sorbic acid Preservative with antibacterial and antifungal properties.

Sorbide nitrate See **Isosorbide dinitrate**.

Sorbitol Carbohydrate poorly absorbed by mouth, but used as intravenous infusion it is a useful source of calories. May also be used as sweetening agent in diabetic foods, in dialysis fluids, and as a laxative.

Sotalol Beta-adrenoceptor blocking drug. Uses, side effects, etc. as for **Propranolol**.

Soya oil Vegatable oil used intravenously for nutrition in debilitating conditions and topically as an emolient for dry skin. Adverse effects from intravenous use include rash, fever, chills, bone marrow depression, and jaundice.

Spectinomycin Antimicrobial active against a wide range of bacteria. Offers no advantages over other antimicrobials, except in treatment of gonorrhoea where a single injection may be adequate.

Spermicides A number of different substances used in spermicidal contraceptives and administered topically into the vagina as jelly, cream, foaming tablet, pessary, aerosol, or film. Appear to act by reducing surface tension in the sperm cell surface and allowing osmotic imbalance to destroy the cell. Relatively ineffective contraceptives, they should be used in conjunction with a barrier contraceptive (e.g., the cap), unless the couple concerned accept the risk of pregnancy.

Spiramycin Antibiotic with similar actions and adverse effects to **Erythromycin**.

Spironolactone Potassium-sparing diuretic. Acts by antagonism of the sodium-retaining hormone **Aldosterone** and thus prevents exchange of sodium for potassium in the kidney tubule. Diuretic action is weak. Used when **Aldosterone** is an important cause of fluid overload (e.g., liver cirrhosis and nephrotic syndrome). Toxic effects include headache, nausea, vomiting, and swelling of the breasts (especially in men). Danger of excessive potassium retention which,, if severe, is treated with haemodialysis and ion exchange resins.

Squalane Ingredient of skin ointments that increases skin permeability to drugs.

Squill Expectorant. Has irritant action on gastric mucosa and produces reflex expectorant action. Used in cough mixtures for chronic bronchitis when sputum is scanty, but too irritant for use in acute bronchitis. May cause nausea, vomiting, diarrhoea, and slowing of heart rate.

Stanozolol Sex hormone, with actions, uses, and adverse effects similar to **Testosterone**. Long-term use may cause jaundice; used with caution in liver disease.

Starch Polysaccharide prepared from maize, wheat, or potato. Used as an absorbant in dusting powders for skin lesions. Also used as a disintegrating agent in tablets, as a mucilage in infant feeds, and as an antidote in iodine poisoning.

Stearyl alcohol Used in ointments and creams where its solubility aids the incorporation of water or aqueous solution.

Sterculia Plant extract. Takes up moisture and increases faecal mass which promotes peristalsis. Used as a purgative and a bulking agent in treatment of obesity.

Stibocaptate Actions and adverse effects as for **Sodium antimonylgluconate**.

Stibogluconate sodium Antimony derivative. Used in treatment of leishmaniasis. Adverse effects include nausea, vomiting, diarrhoea, muscle and joint pains, and cardiotoxicity.

Stibophen Used in schistosomiasis. Actions and adverse effects as for **Sodium antimonylgluconate**.

Stilboestrol Sex hormone, with actions, uses, and adverse effects similar to **Oestradiol**.

Storax Balsam obtained from trunk of *Liquidambar orientalis*. Has mild antiseptic action. Used topically to assist healing of skin (e.g., for bed sores and nappy rash).

Streptodornase Enzyme derived from streptococcal bacteria. Breaks down proteins in exudates. Used together with **Streptokinase** to help remove clotted blood or fibrinous/purulent accumulations. Administered topically, intramuscularly or by instillation into body cavities (e.g., for haemothorax). May cause pain, fever, nausea, skin rashes, and more severe allergic reactions. If haemorrhage occurs, the treatment is as for **Streptokinase**.

Streptokinase Plasminogen activator/fibrinolytic agent derived from *Streptococcus*. Given intravenously in thrombotic or embolic disease. May produce allergic reactions or haemorrhage which can be reversed by an antifibrinolysin such as **Epsilon-aminocaproic acid** or **Tranexamic acid**.

Streptomycin Bactericidal aminoglycoside antibiotic, active against tubercle bacillus, many gram-negative and some gram-positive organisms. Poorly absorbed orally. Administered intramuscularly. Excreted mainly by kidneys, so accumulates if renal function impaired. Adverse effects include hypersensitivity reactions (particularly contact dermatitis), ototoxicity, and potentiation of neuromuscular blockade.

Strychnine CNS stimulant which is included in small doses in some 'tonics' with no justification. In fact is a potent poison causing convulsions, muscle spasms, coma, and death. Treatment is by prevention of convulsions and assisted respiration.

Styramate Centrally acting muscle relaxant. May cause drowsiness, dizziness, and rashes.

Succinic acid Said to promote absorption of iron from the intestine.

Succinylsulphathiazole Sulphonamide antibacterial, with actions, etc. of **Sulphadimidine**. Poorly absorbed. Used mainly for gut infections and sterilization of bowel prior to surgery.

Sucralfate Aluminium–sucrose complex used for treatment of peptic ulcers. Protects gastro-duodenal mucosa by forming complex with pepsin which adheres to active ulcers. May cause constipation after prolonged use, possibly due to release of aluminium.

Sulconazole Antifungal, with broad spectrum of activity. Used topically for fungal infections of skin (e.g., tinea, pityriasis, and candidiasis). May cause hypersensitivity reactions with itching, burning, redness, and swelling.

Sulfametopyrazine Sulphonamide antibacterial with actions, etc. similar to **Sulphadimidine**. Long-acting. Side effects may be more serious than **Sulphadimidine**.

Sulindac Non-steroid anti-inflammatory agent with actions, uses and adverse effects similar to **Ibuprofen**.

Sulphacarbamide Sulphonamide antibacterial, with actions and adverse effects similar to **Sulphadimidine**. Rapidly excreted in urine and therefore used for urinary tract infections. Crystalluria said not to occur.

Sulphacetamide Sulphonamide antibacterial, with actions similar to **Sulphadimidine**, but used only as eye drops for eye infections.

Sulphadiazine Sulphonamide antibacterial, with actions, etc. similar to **Sulphadimidine**.

Sulphadimethoxine Sulphonamide antibacterial, with actions, etc. of **Sulphadimidine**, but only once daily administration required.

Sulphadimidine Sulphonamide antibacterial, which inhibits conversion of *para*-**Aminobenzoic acid** to **Folic acid**. Broad spectrum of activity. Mainly used in urinary tract infections. Adverse effects include crystalluria, skin rashes, polyarteritis, and Stevens–Johnson syndrome. May produce kernicterus in newborn. Potentiates **Warfarin** by competitive displacement from plasma proteins.

Sulphafurazole Sulphonamide antibacterial, with actions, etc. similar to **Sulphadimidine**.

Sulphaguanidine Sulphonamide antibacterial, with actions, etc. of **Sulphadimidine**. Poorly absorbed. Used mainly for gut infections and sterilization of bowel prior to surgery.

Sulphamerazine Sulphonamide antibacterial, with actions, etc. similar to **Sulphadimidine**.

Sulphamethizole Sulphonamide antibacterial, with actions, etc. similar to **Sulphadimidine**.

Sulphamethoxazole Sulphonamide antibacterial, with actions, etc. of **Sulphadimidine**, but somewhat longer action.

Sulphamethoxydiazine Sulphonamide antibacterial, with actions, etc. of **Sulphadimidine**, but only once daily administration required.

Sulphamethoxypyridazine Sulphonamide antibacterial, with actions, etc. of **Sulphadimidine**, but only once daily administration required.

Sulphanilamide Sulphonamide antibacterial, with actions and adverse effects similar to **Sulphadimidine** but more toxic. Now used only for topical infections (e.g., in eye or ear drops).

Sulphapyridine Sulphonamide antibacterial, with actions and adverse effects similar to **Sulphadimidine**. Toxic effects are common and its use is generally limited to treatment of dermatitis herpetiformis and other skin conditions.

Sulphasalazine Compound of **Sulphapyridine** and **Salicylic acid** used in ulcerative colitis. Adverse effects as for **Sulphadimidine**.

Sulphasomizole Sulphonamide antibacterial, with actions, etc. of **Sulphadimidine**, but somewhat longer action.

Sulphathiazole Sulphonamide antibacterial, with actions, etc. of **Sulphadimidine**.

Sulphinpyrazone Prophylactic treatment for gout. Promotes renal excretion of urates by reducing reabsorption in renal tubules. Reduces blood uric acid levels and gradually depletes urate deposits in tissues. No value in treatment of acute gout. Reduces platelet stickiness and is used to prevent thrombosis in the coronary and cerebral circulations. May cause nausea, vomiting, and abdominal pain. May aggravate peptic ulcer and may precipitate acute gout. Long-term use may suppress bone marrow activity. Caution in renal disease and peptic ulcer. May interact to enhance actions of oral anticoagulants and oral hypoglycaemics.

Sulphormethoxine Sulphonamide antibacterial, with actions, etc. of **Sulphadimidine**, but only once weekly administration required.

Sulphur Used topically in skin lotions or ointments as an antiseptic.

Sulpiride Antipsychotic, with actions (including anti-emetic) and uses similar to **Chlorpromazine**. Adverse effects include sedation, extrapyramidal symptoms, sleep disturbance, agitation, and hypertension.

Sulthiame Anticonvulsant. Carbonic anhydrase inhibitor similar to **Acetazolamide**. Used in prevention of epilepsy, usually in addition to other drugs. May cause paraesthesia of face and extremities, hyperventilation, and gastric upsets. Inhibits **Phenytoin** metabolism and may cause phenytoin toxicity. In overdosage causes vomiting, headache, hyperventilation, and vertigo but not coma. May cause crystalluria with renal damage which is treated by alkaline diuresis.

Suprofen Non-steroid anti-inflammatory analgesic with actions, uses and adverse effects similar to **Ibuprofen**.

Suramin Anti-worm treatment. Used in filiariasis. May cause impairment of kidney function. Use reserved for cases resistant to less toxic drugs.

Suxamethonium Muscle relaxant. Acts by depolarization of muscle end plate, rendering the tissue incapable of responding to the neurotransmitter. Action limited by destruction by pseudocholinesterase. Used as an adjunct to anaesthesia for surgery. Short-acting, but effects are prolonged in patients with reduced pseudocholinesterase levels. May cause bradycardia, cardiac arrhythmias, fever, and bronchospasm. Prolonged respiratory paralysis is treated by assisted ventilation and *not* by anticholinesterases.

T

Talampicillin Antimicrobial ester of **Ampicillin** to which it is rapidly metabolized after absorption. Uses and adverse effects similar to **Ampicillin**. Said to maintain higher blood levels and to cause less diarrhoea.

Talc Has lubricant and anti-irritant properties. Used topically on skin and as an aid to the manufacture of some tablets.

Tamoxifen Antioestrogen. Competes with oestrogen for tissue receptor sites. Used as palliative treatment for breast cancer and in treatment of infertility due to failure of ovulation. May cause gastro-intestinal disturbance, fluid retention, hot flushes, and vaginal bleeding.

Tannic acid Astringent. Precipitates proteins and forms complexes with some heavy metals and alkaloids. May be used topically on skin for minor burns, abrasions or chilblains. Formerly used orally to reduce absorption of some poisons. May cause liver damage, nausea, and vomiting.

Tartrazine Orange-coloured dye. Used to colour some foods and medicines. May cause hypersensitivity reactions. Shows cross-sensitivity with **Acetylsalicylic acid**.

Temazepam Benzodiazepine tranquillizer/hypnotic similar to **Nitrazepam**, but with shorter duration of action and therefore less tendency to impair CNS function on the following day.

Terbutaline Beta-adrenoceptor agonist. Actions, uses, and adverse effects as for **Salbutamol**.

Terebene Pleasant-smilling oil used to mask unpleasant odours or tastes and as a vapour to relieve nasal decongestion. Large doses are irritant to the gastro-intestinal tract.

Terfenadine Antihistamine, with actions and adverse effects similar to **Promethazine** but is claimed to produce less sedation. Used for hay fever and allergic skin conditions.

Terlipressin Prodrug which, after injection, is converted in the body into **Vasopressin**.

Testosterone Male sex hormone. Controls development and maintenance of male sex hormones and secondary sex characteristics (androgenic effects). Also produces metabolic effects that lead to increased growth of bone, water retention, increased production of red blood cells, and increased blood vessel formation in the skin (anabolic effects). Used in the male to speed sexual development, but of no value in treating sterility or impotence unless related to sexual underdevelopment. In the female used to treat some menstrual disorders, for suppression of lactation, and to reduce growth of breast tumours. Has also been used for anabolic effects in debilitated patients, but now superseded by new drugs. Unwanted effects include excess fluid and water retention, stimulation of growth of prostate tumours, and virilization in females.

Tetrabenazine Used to suppress abnormal movements (e.g., Huntington's chorea). Adverse effects include drowsiness, gastro-intestinal upsets, and depression.

Tetrachloroethylene Used in treatment of hookworms. Adverse effects include nausea, vomiting, diarrhoea, and vertigo.

Tetracosactrin Synthetic polypeptide, with actions, uses, and adverse effects similar to **Corticotrophin**. Used intravenously as a test of adrenal function or by depot injection for treatment of inflammatory or degenerative disorders.

Tetracycline Bacteriostatic antibiotic, active against many gram-positive and gram-negative organisms, some viruses and chlamydia. Adverse effects include diarrhoea and *Candida* bowel superinfection, yellow discoloration of teeth, inhibition of bone growth in children, and exacerbation of renal failure. Interacts in the bowel with compounds of iron, calcium, and aluminium to produce insoluble chelates that are not absorbed.

Tetranicotinoylfructose Peripheral vasodilator with actions similar to **Nicotinic acid**. Used to treat reduced peripheral circulation (e.g., Raynaud's syndrome). May cause flushing, rashes, and heavy menstrual blood losses.

Thenyldiamine Antihistamine, with actions, uses, and adverse effects similar to **Promethazine** but shorter duration of action.

Theobromine Xanthine derivative. No useful CNS stimulant effects. Has been used as a diuretic or to dilate coronary or peripheral arteries. Now superseded by more effective agents but still found in some mixtures.

Theophylline May be used as a bronchodilator, but **Aminophylline** and other derivatives are more commonly used as bronchial muscle relaxants.

Theophylline ethylenediamine See **Aminophylline**.

Thiabendazole Used in treatment of roundworms. Adverse effects include nausea, drowsiness, and vertigo.

Thiamine See Aneurine.

Thiazides A group of related compounds. (e.g., **Bendrofluazide**), with diuretic effects. They act at the distal convulated tubule of the kidney to reduce reabsorption of salt and water. Moderately potent, but less so than the 'loop diuretics' (e.g., **Frusemide**). Active by mouth within one to two hours and a duration of 12–24 hours. May cause hypokalaemia, hyperglycaemia, and hyperuricaemia. Caution in patients with diabetes mellitus and gout. Used as diuretics where they act partly by reducing the peripheral vascular resistance.

Thiethylperazine Phenothiazine with actions similar to **Chlorpromazine** but little tranquillizing effect. Used as an anti-emetic. Given orally, by injection or as suppository. Adverse effects, etc. as for **Chlorpromazine**.

Thioacetazone Anti-tuberculous agent, used as a cheap alternative to *para*-**Aminosalicylic acid**. May cause gastro-intestinal symptoms, blurred vision, conjunctivitis, and allergic reactions.

Thioguanine Cytotoxic drug, with actions, uses, and adverse effects similar to **Mercaptopurine**.

Thiomersal Mercurial disinfectant, with antibacterial and antifungal actions. Used topically to prepare skin for operation. Also used in eye drops and for urethral irrigation. May cause hypersensitivity rashes.

Thiopentone sodium Very short-acting barbiturate used intravenously for anaesthesia of short duration or induction of anaesthesia prior to use of other anaesthetics. Mode of action and adverse effects similar to **Amylobarbitone**.

Thiopropazate Phenothiazine tranquillizer, with actions, uses, etc. similar to **Chlorpromazine**.

Thioridazine Phenothiazine tranquillizer similar to **Chlorpromazine**. Used in treatment of psychoses, confusion, and agitation.

Thio-TEPA Cytotoxic drug used in neoplastic disease. Adverse effects include bone marrow depression.

Thiothixene Tranquillizer essentially similar to **Chlorpromazine**.

Thonzylamine Antihistamine, with actions, uses, and adverse effects similar to **Promethazine** but shorter duration of action.

Threitol dimethane sulphonate Cytotoxic drug used for treatment of ovarian cancer. May cause gastro-intestinal disturbance, bone marrow suppression, and allergic rashes.

Thromboplastin Blood-clotting factor, usually extracts of cattle brains, used in a test that measures blood coagulability.

Thymol Disinfectant, similar to but less toxic than **Phenol**. Used in mouth washes.

Thymoxamine Alpha-adrenoceptor blocking drug used in peripheral vascular disease and glaucoma. Produces sedation and nasal stuffiness on intravenous administration.

Thyrotrophin Pituitary hormone that stimulates production of thyroid hormones. Used in tests of thyroid function.

Thyroxine Thyroid hormone. Has a stimulating action in general metabolism which is delayed in onset and prolonged (see **Liothyronine**). Used in treatment of thyroid deficiency. Doses in excess of requirements may cause thyrotoxic symptoms (e.g., rapid pulse, cardiac arrhythmias, diarrhoea, anxiety features, sweating, weight loss, and muscular weakness). Caution if there is pre-existing heart disease.

Tiaprofenic acid Non-steroid anti-inflammatory/analgesic, with actions, uses, and adverse effects similar to **Ibuprofen**.

Ticarcillin Broad-spectrum **Penicillin** injection reserved for the treatment of severe, life-threatening infections. Dosage must be reduced in the presence of severe renal impairment. Adverse effects similar to other **Penicillins**.

Tigloidine Chemically similar to **Atropine**, but lacks most anticholinergic effects. Recommended for treatment of muscular rigidity and spasticity.

Timolol Beta-adrenoceptor blocking drug. Uses and adverse effects as for **Propranolol**, but mainly used by local conjunctival instillation as eyedrops for glaucoma and orally to prevent recurrence of myocardial infarction.

Tinidazole Antimicrobial used for prevention of postoperative anaerobic, and acute gum infections. May cause nausea, vomiting, and bone marrow suppression.

Titanium dioxide Dermatological treatment. Reduces itching and absorbs ultraviolet rays. Used topically to prevent sunburn and to treat some forms of eczema.

Tobramycin Antimicrobial. Actions and adverse effects similar to **Gentamicin**.

Tocainide Cardiac antiarrhythmic drug with actions similar to **Lignocaine**, but active after oral administration. May cause blood dyscrasias in long-term use. Reserved for acute life-threatening arrhythmias.

Tolazamide Antidiabetic, with actions, uses, and adverse effects similar to **Chlorpropamide**.

Tolazoline Alpha-adrenoceptor blocking drug with partial agonist activity and smooth muscle relaxant properties. Used in peripheral vascular disease. Side effects include flushing, tachycardia, nausea, and vomiting.

Tolbutamide Oral antidiabetic drug, with actions, uses, and adverse effects similar to **Chlorpropamide**, but excreted more rapidly and thus shorter-acting. Recommended when there is greater danger of hypoglycaemia (e.g., in the elderly).

Tolmetin Non-steroid anti-inflammatory/analgesic, with actions, uses, and adverse effects similar to **Ibuprofen**.

Tolnaftate Antifungal agent used as cream or powder for skin infections.

Tolu Balsam obtained from trunk of *Myroxylon balsamum*. Used in cough mixtures for expectorant action and flavour.

Tragacanth Purgative. Increases faecal bulk by the same mechanism as **Methylcellulose**. Occasionally causes allergic rashes or asthma.

Tramazoline Sympathomimetic agent used topically as nasal decongestant. Actions and adverse effects similar to **Naphazoline**.

Tranexamic acid Antifibrinolytic agent, used to reverse effects of **Streptokinase** or other fibrinolytic activity.

Tranylcypromine Antidepressant. Inhibits monoamine oxidase. Actions and adverse effects similar to **Phenelzine**, but less likely to cause hepatitis. Also has **Amphetamine**-like properties.

Trazodone Antidepressant. Blocks neuronal uptake of 5-hydroxytryptamine (serotonin). Unlike the tricyclic antidepressants (e.g., **Amitriptyline**) does not have anticholinergic properties. Thus, tends to be better tolerated in dose and overdose. Adverse effects include gastric discomfort, dry mouth, headache, dizziness, drowsiness, insomnia, and slight hypotension.

Treosulfan Cytotoxic drug, used in treatment of ovarian cancer. Metabolized by liver to active, epoxide form. Acts by damaging DNA and thus interfering with cell replication. Adverse effects include gastro-intestinal symptoms, skin reactions, hair loss, and bone marrow depression.

Tretinoin **Vitamin A** derivative. Used topically in some dermatological treatments (e.g., for acne).

Triamcinolone Potent synthetic **Corticosteroid**, with actions, etc. similar to **Cortisone**. Used mainly for topical treatment of certain skin rashes (e.g., eczema).

Triamterene Potassium-sparing diuretic similar to **Amiloride**.

Triazolam Benzodiazepine tranquillizer/hypnotic, with actions, uses, and adverse effects similar to **Nitrazepam**.

Trichloroethylene Weak inhalational anaesthetic with good analgesic but poor muscle relaxant properties. Used mostly in short surgical procedures (e.g., in obstetrics). May slow the heart and lead to irregular rhythms. Anaesthesia is sometimes followed by nausea, vomiting and headache. When used as a solution in industry, excessive concentrations may depress liver and kidney function. High concentrations may cause acute poisoning with death in coma.

Trichlorofluoromethane Aerosol propellant/refrigerant. Produces intense cold by its rapid evaporation and thus makes tissues insensitive to pain. Used for relief of muscle pain and spasm.

Triclocarban Disinfectant used in skin preparations and shampoo for prevention/treatment of certain bacterial and fungal infections. Large doses may cause methaemoglobinaemia.

Triclofos Hypnotic/sedative. Hydrolyzed in stomach to trichloroethanol and absorbed as such. More palatable and causes less gastric irritation than **Chloral hydrate** to which it is otherwise similar.

Triclosan Antiseptic solution for pre-operative hand and skin disinfection.

Triethanolamine Emulsifying agent used as ear drops to soften wax for removal. May cause localized skin rashes.

Trifluoperazine Phenothiazine tranquillizer/anti-emetic similar to **Chlorpromazine**.

Trifluperidol Butyrophenone tranquillizer, with actions, uses, and adverse effects similar to **Haloperidol**.

Tri-iodothyronine See **Liothyronine**.

Tri-isopropylphenoxy-polyethoxyethanol Dispersant/emulsifying agent. Used to stabilize oil-in-water mixtures and to disperse and repel spermatozoa thus preventing conception.

Trilostane Used to inhibit synthesis of hormones in the adrenal cortex in conditions such as Cushing's syndrome.

Trimeprazine Phenothiazine similar to **Chlorpromazine**. Used for antiemetic, sedative, and antipruritic effects. Adverse effects, etc. as for **Chlorpromazine**.

Trimetaphan Antihypertensive, with actions and adverse effects similar to **Hexamethonium**, but has very brief duration of action. Used for production of controlled hypotension to reduce blood loss during surgery.

Trimethoprim Antimicrobial. Inhibits conversion of **Folic acid** to **Folinic acid**. Combined with **Sulphamethoxazole** in **Co-trimoxazole**. May also be used on its own for prevention of urinary tract infections. Adverse effects include nausea, vomiting, skin rashes, and bone marrow depression.

Trimipramine Antidepressant, with actions and adverse effects similar to **Amitriptyline**.

Triostam See **Sodium antimonylgluconate**.

Tri-potassium di-citrato bismuthate Bismuth chelate. Used in treatment of peptic ulcer. May cause blackening of the tongue and faeces, constipation, nausea, and vomiting.

Triprolidine Antihistamine, with actions, uses, and adverse effects similar to **Promethazine**.

Tri-sodium edetate Chelating agent, used intravenously in hypercalcaemia and locally for lime burns in the eye. Exchanges sodium ions for calcium ions. May cause nausea, diarrhoea, cramp, and pain in the limb receiving the infusion. Excessive doses may cause renal damage.

Tropicamide Parasympatholytic, used in the eye as a mydriatic and cycloplegic. Actions, etc. similar to **Atropine**, but has rapid onset and short duration of action.

Troxerutin Vitamin derivative claimed to improve strength and reduce permeability of blood vessels. Used to treat haemorrhoids and venous disorders in the legs.

Tryptophan Amino acid, essential component of diet. Converted in the body to 5-hydroxytryptamine (serotonin), a neurotransmitter substance that may be depleted in depression. Used in treatment of depression. May cause nausea, drowsiness and may interact with monoamine oxidase inhibitors (e.g., **Phenelzine**).

Tuberculin Diagnostic agent for tuberculosis. Intradermal injection produces skin reaction in positive cases. May cause skin necrosis in highly sensitive cases.

Tubocurarine Skeletal muscle relaxant. Blocks passage of impulses at the neuromuscular junction. Used as an adjunct to anaesthesia. May cause fall in blood pressure and paralysis of respiration. **Neostigmine** and **Atropine** plus assisted respiration may be used in treatment of toxic effects.

Turmeric Yellow colouring agent with mild spicy flavour, a constituent of curry powder. Included in treatment of 'biliary disorders'.

Turpentine oil Extract of pine used externally as a rubefacient. May cause rashes and vomiting. Rarely used internally but acts as an evacuant if given rectally.

Tyloxapol Mucolytic. Administered by inhalation from a nebulizer. Liquefies mucus and aids expectoration where viscid mucus is troublesome (e.g., chronic bronchitis). May cause inflammation of eyelids. If left open, the solution is prone to bacterial infections.

Tyrothricin Antimicrobial. Too toxic for systemic use but used for topical treatment of skin, mouth, or ear infections.

U

Undecenoic acid Antifungal. Applied topically to skin [e.g., in treatment of tinea pedis (athlete's foot)].

Urea Osmotic diuretic, with actions and uses similar to **Mannitol**. May cause gastric irritation with nausea and vomiting. Intravenous use may cause fall in blood pressure and venous thrombosis at site of injection. Largely superseded by **Mannitol** and other diuretics. Topically in a cream it is used to reduce excess scaling (ichthyosis) and soften the skin.

Urea hydrogen peroxide Disinfectant/deodorant used as a source of **Hydrogen peroxide**.

Urethane Cytotoxic drug. Used in treatment of certain neoplastic diseases but largely superseded by newer drugs. May cause gastro-intestinal disturbance and bone marrow depression. Has also mild hypnotic properties and is used as an anaesthetic for small animals.

Urofollitrophin Follicle-stimulating hormone that stimulates ovulation, extracted from human post-menopausal urine.

Urokinase Enzyme produced by the kidney and excreted in urine. Like **Streptokinase**, it activates plasminogen and is used intravenously to break down blood clots in pulmonary embolism. Adverse effects and their treatment similar to **Streptokinase**.

Ursodeoxycholic acid Used to aid dissolution of cholesterol gall stones. May produce diarrhoea.

V

Valerian CNS depressant occasionally used for sedative effects. No advantage over other drugs that are in more common usage.

Vancomycin Antibiotic, used in infections with **Penicillin**-resistant staphylococci. Must be given intravenously. Adverse effects include ototoxicity.

Vasopressin Posterior pituitary hormone. Has antidiuretic action on kidney and constricts peripheral blood vessels. Used by injection in diagnosis and treatment of diabetes insipidus. May be used to control bleeding from oesophageal varices. May cause pallor, nausea, eructations, cramps, and angina.

Vecuronium Skeletal muscle relaxant with uses and adverse effects similar to **Tubocurarine**.

Verapamil Used in prevention of angina of effort, hypertension, and in treatment of cardiac dysrhythmias. May cause nausea, dizziness and fall in blood pressure. Contraindicated in heart failure.

Veratrum Natural product. Reduces sympathetic tone. Was used in hypertension, but seldom now because of adverse effects which include nausea, vomiting, sweats, dizziness, respiratory depression, and abnormal heart rhythms.

Vidarabine Antiviral agent, with actions, adverse effects similar to **Cytarabine**.

Viloxazine Antidepressant with some anticonvulsant properties. Unlike the tricyclic antidepressants (e.g., **Imipramine**), it is said to have no anticholinergic or sedative properties. Used in treatment of depression, especially when those effects occur from other drugs. May cause nausea and vomiting. If given with **Phenytoin** may induce toxicity due to that drug. No antidote; overdosage treated symptomatically.

Vinblastine Cytotoxic alkaloid from West Indian periwinkle, used in neoplastic disease. Adverse effects include neuropathy and bone marrow depression.

Vincristine Cytotoxic, with actions and adverse effects as for **Vinblastine**.

Vindesine Semisynthetic cytotoxic derived from **Vinblastine**. Has a broader spectrum of antitumour activity than the parent compound and apparently does not share cross-resistance with **Vinblastine** or **Vincristine**. Used mainly for leukaemia and malignant melanoma. Adverse effects include haematological, neurological, cutaneous, and gastro-intestinal effects.

Viomycin Antibiotic, with actions and adverse effects similar to **Streptomycin**.

Viprynium Used in treatment of threadworms. Adverse effects include red stools, vomiting, and diarrhoea.

Vitamin A Fat-soluble vitamin present in liver, dairy products, and some vegetables, essential for normal visual function and for maintenance of epithelial surfaces. Overdosage produces mental changes, hyperkeratosis, and hypoprothrombinaemia.

Vitamin B_1 See **Aneurine**.

Vitamin B_2 See **Riboflavine**.

Vitamin B_6 See **Pyridoxine**.

Vitamin B_7 See **Nicotinic acid**.

Vitamin B_{12} See **Hydroxocobalamin**.

Vitamin C (Ascorbic acid) Vitamin found in fruit and vegetables, necessary for normal collagen formation. Deficiency causes scurvy with mucosal bleeding and anaemia. High-dose administration in prophylaxis against common cold is controversial. Similarly, although vitamin C influences the formation of haemaglobin and red cell maturation, its addition to haematinics is of questionable value for most patients.

Vitamin D (Calciferol) Group of fat-soluble vitamins found in dairy products and formed in skin exposed to sunlight. Promotes gut absorption of calcium and its mobilization from bone. Deficiency produces rickets and bone softening. Excess produces hypercalcaemia, ectopic calcification, and renal failure.

Vitamin E (Tocopheryl) Vitamin with no clearly defined requirements or deficiency disease in man. Has been suggested as treatment for habitual abortion, cardiovascular disease, and other conditions.

Vitamin K (Menaphthone, Menadiol, Phytomenadione, Acetomenaphthone) Fat-soluble vitamin responsible for formation of prothrombin and other clotting factors. Used to reverse oral anticoagulants and in bleeding diseases. Excessive dosing may produce haemolysis.

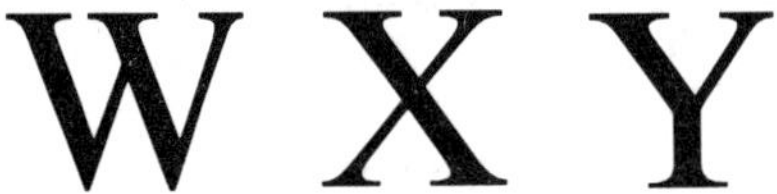

Warfarin Coumarin anticoagulant that interferes with synthesis of clotting factors by the liver. May produce allergic reactions. Overdosage produces haemorrhage controlled by **Vitamin K**. Potentiated by drugs such as **Acetylsalicylic acid** and **Phenylbutazone** which displace from protein binding, and reduced by hepatic enzyme inducers, such as barbiturates. Caution if used in liver disease.

Wheat husk Concentrated extract of non-absorbable fibre content of wheat. Used as bulking agent in treatment of constipation. May cause flatulence and abdominal distension.

Wool fat Fat/grease recovered from wool. Resembles the secretion from human sebaceous glands in the skin. Mixed with vegetable or soft paraffin oils it produces emollient creams which penetrate the skin and aid drug absorption through the skin. May cause skin sensitization.

Xipamide Diuretic with potency similar to **Frusemide** but slower onset and longer duration of action. Uses and adverse effects similar to **Bendrofluazide**.

Xylometazoline Sympathomimetic, used topically as nasal decongestant. Actions and adverse effects similar to **Naphazoline**.

Yohimbine Plant extract with alpha-adrenoceptor blocking actions. Said to have aphrodisiac properties but not proven.

Z

Zinc chloride Astringent/deodorant. Used in mouth wash and for application to wounds. Caustic in higher concentrations.

Zinc ichthammol Mixture of **Zinc oxide** and **Ichthammol** used for treatment of eczema.

Zinc naphthenate Used topically for fungal infections of the skin.

Zinc oleate Topical treatment for eczema. Actions similar to **Zinc oxide**.

Zinc oxide Dermatological treatment. Has mild astringent, soothing, and protective effects. Used topically in treatment of eczema and excoriated skin.

Zinc phenolsulphonate Antiseptic dusting powder similar to **Zinc oxide**.

Zinc powder See **Zinc oxide**.

Zinc salicylate Dermatological treatment, with actions and uses similar to **Zinc oxide**.

Zinc sulphate Astringent used topically for skin wounds/ulcers to assist healing. Also included in some eye drops for minor allergic conjunctivitis. Orally it is an emetic, but is not used for this purpose due to toxic effects. In smaller, sustained release doses, it is used for nutritional zinc deficiency. For zinc-deficiency states, a soluble formulation causes less gastro-intestinal disturbance.

Zinc undecenoate Antifungal used topically for fungal infections of the skin.

Zimelidine Antidepressant, with actions, uses, and adverse effects similar to **Trazadone**. Withdrawn in 1984 due to adverse effects including peripheral neuropathy.

Zomepirac Anti-inflammatory analgesic, with actions, uses, and adverse effects similar to **Ibuprofen**. Now withdrawn.

Part II

Trade Names

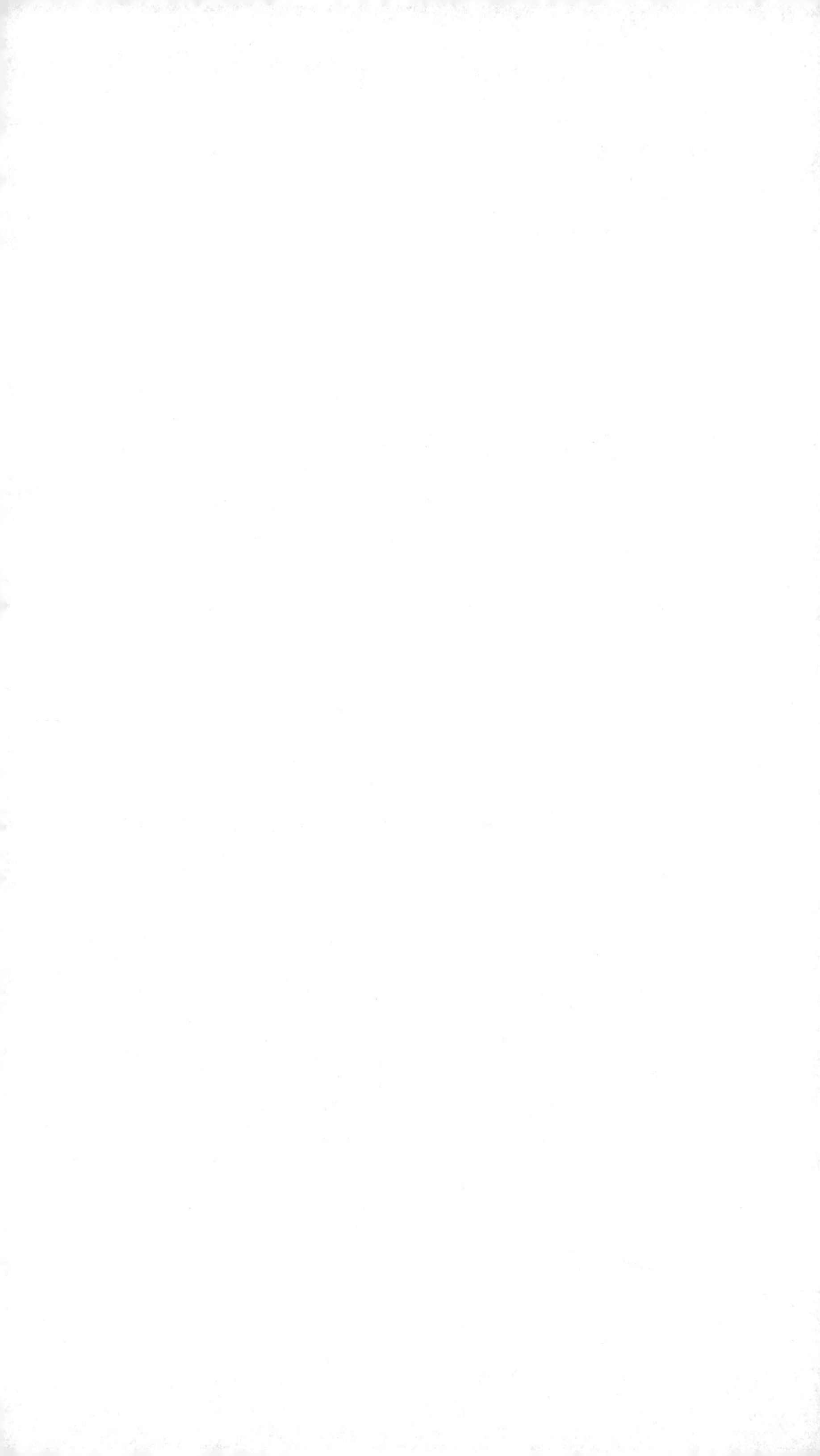

A

AAA Mouth and Throat Spray. Local anaesthetic/antiseptic for sore throat: see **Benzocaine, Cetalkonium**.
Abicol. Antihypertensive: see **Bendrofluazide, Reserpine**.
Abidec. Vitamin mixture: see **Aneurine, Riboflavine, Vitamin A, Vitamin D**.
Acepril. Antihypertensive: see **Captopril**.
Acetoxyl. Topical gel for treatment of acne: see **Benzoyl peroxide**.
Achromycin. Anti-infective. See **Tetracycline**.
Acidol-Pepsin. Acid/pepsin mixture for use in achlorhydria.
Aci-Jel. Jelly for topical treatment of vaginal infection.
Acnegel. Topical gel for treatment of acne: see **Benzoyl peroxide**.
Acnil. Topical treatment for acne: see **Cetrimide, Resorcinol**.
Actal. Antacid: see **Alexitol sodium**.
Acthar gel. Corticotrophic hormone injection: see **Corticotrophin**.
Actidil. Antihistamine: see **Triprolidine**.
Actifed. Decongestant: see **Pseudoephedrine, Triprolidine**.
Actifed Compound Linctus. As Actifed plus **Dextromethorphan** for cough suppression.
Actinac. Topical treatment for acne: see **Chloramphenicol, Hydrocortisone**.
Actonorm. Antacid: see **Aluminium hydroxide, Magnesium hydroxide, Simethicone**.
Actrapid MC. Purified crystalline pork insulin: see **Insulin**.
Acupan. Analgesic: see **Nefopam**.
Adalat. Antianginal: see **Nifedipine**.
Adalat retard. Sustained-release vasodilator antihypertensive: see **Nifedipine**.
Adcortyl. Corticosteroid for topical or systemic use: see **Triamcinolone**.
Addamel. Electrolytes and trace elements for parenteral nutrition.
Addiphos. Source of phosphate during parenteral feeding.
Adriamycin. Cytotoxic antibiotic: see **Doxorubicin**.
Aerosporin. Antibiotic: see **Polymyxin B**.
Aerrane. General anaesthetic: see **Isoflurane**.
Afrazine. Nasal decongestant: see **Oxymetazoline**.
Agarol. Laxative: see **Liquid paraffin, Phenolphthalein**.
Agiolax. Purgative: see **Ispaghula, Sennoside B**.
Aglutella Gentili (b). **Gluten**-free pasta, low in protein, sodium, and potassium. Dietary substitute used in chronic renal failure and phenylketonuria.
Airbron. Mucolytic: see **Acetylcysteine**.

Akrotherm. Topical treatment for chilblains: see **Acetylcholine, Histamine**.
Alavac. Vaccines for desensitization to pollens and other allergens in asthma and hay fever.
Albay. Injection of bee venom extract for desensitization of allergic individuals: see **Allergen extract vaccines**.
Albucid. Anti-infective eye drops: see **Sulphacetamide**.
Albumaid Preps (b). Range of dietary substitutes for use in malabsorption and inherited metabolic disorders (e.g., phenylketonuria).
Alcobon. Antifungal for systemic yeast infections: see **Flucytosine**.
Alcoderm. Emollient cream/lotion for protection of dry skin: see **Cetyl alcohol, Ethanolamine, Liquid Paraffin, Polysorbate 60, Sodium lauryl sulphate, Stearyl alcohol**.
Alcomicin. Antibiotic eye drops: see **Gentamicin**.
Alcopar. Anthelmintic: see **Bephenium**.
Alcos-Anal. Local anaesthetic for haemorrhoids: see **Chlorothymol, Sodium morrhuate**.
Aldactide. Diuretic/antihypertensive: see **Hydroflumethiazide, Spironolactone**.
Aldactone. Diuretic: see **Spironolactone**.
Aldomet. Antihypertensive: see **Methyldopa**.
Alembicol D (b). Lipid extract of coconut oil; substitute for long-chain fats in fat malabsorption.
Aleudrin. Sympathomimetic bronchodilator: see **Isoprenaline**.
Alevaire. Mucolytic: see **Tyloxapol**.
Alexan. Cytotoxic: see **Cytarabine**.
Algesal. Rubefacient: see **Diethylamine salicylate**.
Algipan. Rubefacient: see **Capsicum, Histamine, Nicotinic acid, Salicylic acid**.
Alka-Donna. Antacid: see **Aluminium hydroxide, Belladonna extract, Magnesium trisilicate**.
Alkeran. Cytotoxic: see **Melphalan**.
Allbee with C. Vitamin supplement: see **Aneurine, Nicotinic acid, Pantothenic acid, Pyridoxine, Riboflavine, Vitamin C**.
Allegron. Antidepressant: see **Nortriptyline**.
Alloferin. Muscle relaxant: see **Alcuronium**.
Allpyral. Desensitizing vaccines similar to Alavac.
Almazine. Anxiolytic: see **Lorazepam**.
Almevax. Live attenuated **Rubella vaccine**.
Alophen. Purgative: see **Aloin, Belladonna extract, Ipecacuanha, Phenolphthalein**.
Aloral. For gout: see **Allopurinol**.
Alphaderm. Topical corticosteroid cream: see **Hydrocortisone, Urea**.
Alpha Keri Bath. Emollient bath additive for dry skin: see **Liquid paraffin, Wool fat**.
Alphosyl. Topical treatments for psoriasis and other scaly disorders: see **Allantoin, Coal tar**.

Alphosyl HC. Topical steroid treatment for psoriasis: see **Allantoin, Coal tar, Hydrocortisone**.
Alrheumat. Non-steroid anti-inflammatory: see **Ketoprofen**.
Altacaps. Antacid: see **Dimethicone, Hydrotalcite**.
Altacite. Antacid: see **Hydrotalcite**.
Alu-Cap. Antacid: see **Aluminium hydroxide**.
Aludrox. Antacid: see **Aluminium hydroxide**.
Aludrox SA. Antacid/sedative: see **Aluminium hydroxide, Ambutonium, Magnesium hydroxide**.
Aluhyde. Antacid/antispasmodic: see **Aluminium hydroxide, Belladonna extract, Magnesium trisilicate**.
Aluline. For gout: see **Allopurinol**.
Alunex. Anti-allergic: see **Chlorpheniramine**.
Alupent. Sympathomimetic bronchodilator: see **Orciprenaline**.
Alupent expectorant. Bronchodilator/mucolytic: see **Bromhexine, Orciprenaline**.
Alupram. Anxiolytic: see **Diazepam**.
Aluzine. Diuretic: see **Frusemide**.
Aluzyme. Vitamin mixture: see **Aneurine, Folic acid, Nicotinic acid, Riboflavine**.
Alyrane. General anaesthetic: see **Enflurane**.
Ambaxin. Antibiotic: see **Bacampicillin**.
Ambihar. Antiworm: see **Niridazole**.
Amesec. Bronchodilator: see **Aminophylline, Ephedrine**.
Amfipen. Antibiotic: see **Ampicillin**.
Amikin. Antibiotic: see **Amikacin**.
Amilco. Diuretic combination: see **Amiloride, Hydrochlorothiazide**.
Amin-ex biscuits (b). Low **Amino acids**/protein dietary substitute for use in phenylketonuria and renal failure.
Aminofusin L600 and L1000. Solutions of **Amino acids** for intravenous feeding.
Aminogran (b). Low **Amino acids** food substitute for phenylketonuria.
Aminoplasmal. Intravenous **Amino acids** and electrolytes for parenteral nutrition.
Aminoplex 5 and 14. Intravenous **Amino acids, Sorbitol**, ethanol, vitamins and electrolytes.
Amisyn. Peripheral vasodilator: see **Acetomenaphthone, Nicotinamide**.
Amoxil. Antibiotic: see **Amoxycillin**.
Ampiclox. Antibiotic: see **Ampicillin, Cloxacillin**.
Amsidine. Cytotoxic: see **Amsacrine**.
Amytal (c). Hypnotic/minor tranquillizer: see **Amylobarbitone**.
Anacal. Topical treatment for haemorrhoids: see **Hexachlorophane, Prednisolone**.
Anaflex lozenges. Antiseptic for mouth and throat: see **Polynoxylin**.
Anaflex topical preps. Skin antiseptic: see **Polynoxylin**.
Anafranil. Antidepressant: see **Clomipramine**.
Ananase forte. Proteolytic enzymes for post-traumatic tissue reactions.
Anapolon. Anabolic steroid: see **Oxymetholone**.

Ancoloxin. Anti-emetic: see **Meclozine, Pyridoxine**.
Androcur. For male sexual disorders: see **Cyproterone**.
Andursil. Antacid: see **Aluminium hydroxide, Dimethicone, Magnesium carbonate, Magnesium hydroxide**.
Anectine. Muscle relaxant during anaesthesia: see **Suxamethonium**.
Anethaine. Topical anaesthetic for haemorrhoids: see **Amethocaine**.
Aneurone. Tonic. Traditional remedy for loss of appetite: see **Caffeine, Compound gentian infusion, Sodium acid phosphate, Strychnine, Thiamine**.
Angilol. Beta-adrenoceptor blocker: see **Propranolol**.
Anhydrol forte. Antiperspirant: see **Aluminium chloride**.
Anodesyn. Local treatment for haemorrhoids: see **Allantoin, Bronopol, Ephedrine, Lignocaine**.
Anovlar 21. Oral contraceptive: see **Ethinyloestradiol, Norethisterone**.
Anquil. Tranquillizer: see **Benperidol**.
Antabuse. For treatment of alcoholism: see **Disulfiram**.
Antasil. Antacid: see **Aluminium hydroxide, Dimethicone, Magnesium hydroxide**.
Antepar. For threadworms and roundworms: see **Piperazine**.
Antepsin. Mucosal protective for treatment of peptic ulceration: see **Sucralfate**.
Anthical. Antihistamine cream for skin inflammation: see **Mepyramine, Zinc oxide**. May cause skin rash.
Anthisan cream. Antihistamine for insect bites: see **Mepyramine**.
Anthisan elixir. Antihistamine for allergy: see **Mepyramine**.
Anthranol. Topical ointment for psoriasis: see **Dithranol, Salicylic acid**.
Antisin-Privine. Anti-allergic nasal decongestant: see **Antazoline, Naphazoline**.
Antoin. Analgesic: see **Acetylsalicylic acid, Caffeine, Calcium carbonate, Codeine**.
Antraderm. For treatment of psoriasis: see **Dithranol**.
Anturan. Increases urate excretion in gout: see **Sulphinpyrazone**.
Anugesic-HC. Topical treatment for haemorrhoids: see **Benzyl benzoate, Hydrocortisone, Pramoxine, Zinc oxide**.
Anusol. Local treatment for haemorrhoids: see **Benzyl benzoate, Bismuth subgallate, Bismuth oxide, Zinc oxide**.
Anusol HC. As Anusol plus **Hydrocortisone**.
Anxon. Anxiolytic: see **Ketazolam**.
Apisate (c). Anti-obesity: see **Aneurine, Diethylpropion**.
APP. Antacid/anticholinergic for gastro-intestinal disorders: see **Aluminium hydroxide, Calcium carbonate, Homatropine, Magnesium carbonate, Papaverine**.
Apresoline. Antihypertensive: see **Hydralazine**.
Aprinox. Diuretic: see **Bendrofluazide**.
Aproten (b). **Gluten**-free products for coeliac disease.
Apsifen. Non-steroid anti-inflammatory/analgesic: see **Ibuprofen**.
Apsin V.K. Antibiotic: see **Phenoxymethylpenicillin**.
Apsolol. Beta-adrenoceptor blocker: see **Propranolol**.

Apsolox. Beta-adrenoceptor blocker: see **Oxprenolol**.
Aquadrate. Keratolytic for thickened, dry skin: see **Urea**.
Aradolene. Rubefacient: see **Salicylate**.
Aramine. Vasoconstrictor for shock: see **Metaraminol**.
Arelix. Diuretic: see **Piretanide**.
Arfonad. Hypotensive: see **Trimetaphan**.
Argotone. Nasal decongestant: see **Ephedrine, Silver protein**.
Arilvax. Vaccine for immunization against yellow fever.
Arobon. Antidiarrhoeal: see **Ceratonia, Starch**.
Arpicolin. Syrup formulation. Anticholinergic/antiparkinsonian: see **Procyclidine**.
Arpimycin. Antibiotic: see **Erythromycin**.
Arret. Antidiarrhoeal: see **Loperamide**.
Artane. Antiparkinsonian/anticholinergic: see **Benzhexol**.
Artracin. Non-steroid anti-inflammatory/analgesic: see **Indomethacin**.
Arvin. Anticoagulant: see **Ancrod**.
Asacol. For ulcerative colitis: see **Mesalazine**.
Ascabiol. Topical treatment for scabies and lice: see **Benzyl benzoate**.
Ascalix. Antiworm: see **Piperazine**.
Aserbine. Desloughing cream/solution for removal of clots and slough in wounds or ulcers: see **Benzoic acid, Hexachlorophane, Malic acid, Propylene glycol, Salicylic acid**.
Asilone. Antacid: see **Aluminium hydroxide, Dimethicone**.
Asmapax. For asthma: see **Ephedrine, Theophylline**.
Asmaven. Sympathomimetic bronchodilator: see **Salbutamol**.
Asma-Vydrin. Inhalation for asthma: see **Adrenaline, Atropine methonitrate, Papaverine**.
Aspav. Water-dispersable, analgesic tablets: see **Acetylsalicylic acid, Papaveretum**.
Aspellin. Rubefacient: see **Acetylsalicylic acid, Methyl salicylate**.
Aspergum. Analgesic/antipyretic chewing gum: see **Acetylsalicylic acid**.
Astiban. For treatment of schistosomiasis: see **Stibocaptate**.
A.T. 10. For Vitamin D deficiency or resistance: see **Dihydrotachysterol**.
Atarax. Sedative/tranquillizer: see **Hydroxyzine**.
Atensine. Sedative/tranquillizer: see **Diazepam**.
Ativan. Sedative/tranquillizer: see **Lorazepam**.
Atromid-S 500. Antianginal/lipid-lowering agent: see **Clofibrate**.
Atrovent. Bronchodilator for inhalation: see **Ipratropium**.
Attenuvax. Live attenuated **Measles vaccine** with **Neomycin** as antibiotic preservative.
Audax. Drops for middle and outer ear infection: see **Choline salicylate**.
Audicort. Drops for outer ear infection: see **Benzocaine, Neomycin, Triamcinolone**.
Audinorm. Drops for removal of ear wax: see **Dioctylsodium sulphosuccinate, Glycerin**.
Augmentin. Antibacterial: see **Amoxycillin, Clavulanic acid**.
Auralgicin. Drops for middle ear pain: see **Benzocaine, Ephedrine, Phenazone**.

Auraltone. Drops for middle ear pain: see **Benzocaine, Phenazone**.
Aureocort. Topical treatment for allergic/infective skin conditions: see **Chlortetracycline, Triamcinolone**.
Aureomycin. Antibiotic: see **Chlortetracycline**.
Aveeno. For addition to bath for skin allergy.
Aventyl. Antidepressant: see **Nortriptyline**.
Avloclor. Antimalarial: see **Chloroquine**.
Avomine. Antihistamine/anti-emetic: see **Promethazine**.
Azamune. Cytotoxic: see **Azathioprine**.

B

Bacticlens. Antiseptic solution: see **Chlorhexidine**.
Bactigras. Impregnated wound dressing: see **Chlorhexidine**.
Bactrian. Disinfectant cream for skin application: see **Cetrimide**.
Bactrim. Antibacterial: see **Co-trimoxazole**.
Bactroban. Topical antibiotic: see **Mupirocin**.
Balmosa. Rubefacient: see **Benzyl nicotinate, Methyl salicylate**.
Balneum. Topical application for dry skin: see **Soya oil**.
Banocide. For filariasis: see **Diethylcarbamazine**.
Baratol. Antihypertensive: see **Indoramin**.
Barquinol HC. Topical corticosteroid cream for allergic/infectious skin disorders: see **Clioquinol, Hydrocortisone**.
Baxan. Antibiotic: see **Cefadroxil**.
Baycaron. Diuretic: see **Mefruside**.
Bayolin. Rubefacient: see **Glycol salicylate**.
Baypen. Antibiotic: see **Mezlocillin**.
B.C. 500. Vitamin mixture: see **Aneurine, Cyanocobalamin, Nicotinamide, Pantothenic acid, Pyridoxine, Riboflavine, Vitamin C**.
Bebate. Corticosteroid cream for skin application: see **Betamethasone**.
Becloforte. Steroid aerosal for asthma: see **Beclomethasone**.
Beconase. Nasal aerosol for allergic rhinitis: see **Beclomethasone**.
Becosym. Vitamin B complex: see **Aneurine, Nicotinamide, Pyridoxine, Riboflavine**.
Becotide. Steroid aerosol for asthma: see **Beclomethasone**.
Bedranol. Beta-adrenoceptor blocker: see **Propranolol**.
Bellocarb. For reducing gastro-intestinal motility and secretion: see **Belladonna extract, Magnesium trisilicate**.
Benadon. Anti-emetic: see **Pyridoxine**.
Benadryl. Antihistamine for allergy: see **Diphenhydramine**.
Bendogen. Antihypertensive: see **Bethanidine**.
Benemid. Uricosuric for gout: see **Probenecid**.
Benerva. Vitamin for beri-beri and neuritis: see **Aneurine**.
Benerva compound. Vitamin B mixture for deficiency: see **Aneurine, Nicotinamide, Riboflavine**.

Bengue's balsam. Rubefacient: see **Methyl salicylate**.
Benoral. Non-steroid anti-inflammatory/analgesic: see **Benorylate**.
Benoxyl. Topical treatment for acne: see **Benzoyl peroxide**.
Bentex. Antiparkinsonian: see **Benzhexol**.
Benylin. Cough suppressant: see **Diphenhydramine**.
Benylin with codeine. As Benylin with **Codeine**.
Benzagel. Topical gel for treatment of acne: see **Benzoyl peroxide**.
Benztrone. Sex hormone injection for menopausal symptoms and primary amenorrhoea: see **Oestradiol**.
Beogex (d). Purgative: see **Sodium phosphate**.
Berkatens. For treatment of angina, hypertension and arrhythmias: see **Verapamil**.
Berkfurin (d). Urinary anti-infective: see **Nitrofurantoin**.
Berkmycen. Antibiotic: see **Oxytetracycline**.
Berkolol. Beta-adrenoceptor blocker: see **Propranolol**.
Berkozide. Diuretic: see **Bendrofluazide**.
Berotec. Bronchodilator for asthma: see **Fenoterol**.
Beta-Cardone. Beta-adrenoceptor blocker: see **Sotalol**.
Betadine. Antiseptic: see **Providone-iodine**.
Betaloc. Beta-adrenoceptor blocker: see **Metoprolol**.
Betim. Beta-adrenoceptor blocker: see **Timolol**.
Betnelan. Corticosteroid: see **Betamethasone**.
Betnesol. Soluble corticosteroid tablets and injection: see **Betamethasone**.
Betnesol-N. Topical corticosteroid/antibiotic: see **Betamethasone, Neomycin**.
Betnovate. Topical corticosteroid: see **Betamethasone**.
Betnovate C. Topical corticosteroid/anti-infective: see **Betamethasone, Clioquinol**.
Betnovate N. Topical corticosteroid/antibiotic: see **Betamethasone, Neomycin**.
Bextasol inhaler. Steroid aerosol for asthma: see **Betamethasone**.
Bezalip. Lipid-lowering agent: see **Bezafibrate**.
B.F.I. Topical anti-infective powder: see **Bismuth formic iodide, Bismuth subgallate, Boric acid, Zinc phenolsulphonate**.
Bi-Aglut (b). **Gluten**-free biscuits for gluten-sensitive bowel disorders.
Bicillin. Antibiotic: see **Benzylpenicillin, Procaine penicillin**.
BICNU. Cytotoxic: see **Carmustine**.
Bilarcil. Antischistosomiasis: see **Metriphonate**.
Biltricide. Antischistosomiasis: see **Praziquantel**.
Bi Novum. Oral contraceptive: see **Ethinyloestradiol, Norethisterone**.
Biogastrone. For gastric ulcers: see **Carbenoxolone**.
Biomydrin (d). Nasal decongestant/anti-inflammatory: see **Gramicidin, Neomycin, Phenylephrine, Thonzylamine**.
Bioral. Topical therapy for mouth ulcers: see **Carbenoxolone**.
Biorphen. Anticholinergic/antiparkinsonian: see **Orphenadrine**.
Bismodyne. Cream for topical application to relieve pain and irritation from haemorrhoids and other causes of anal discomfort: see **Bismuth subgallate, Hexachlorophane, Lignocaine, Zinc oxide**.

Bisolvomycin. Mucolytic/antibiotic: see **Bromhexine, Oxytetracycline**.
Bisolvon. Mucolytic: see **Bromhexine**.
Bleph-10 (d). Topical antibacterial for eye infections: see **Sulphacetamide**.
Blocadren. Beta-adrenoceptor blocker: see **Timolol**.
Bocasan. Antiseptic mouthwash for oral infections: see **Sodium perborate**.
Bolvidon. Antidepressant: see **Mianserin**.
Bonjela. Topical therapy for mouth ulcers: see **Cetalkonium, Choline salicylate**.
Bradilan. Peripheral vasodilator/lipid-lowering agent: see **Tetranicotinoylfructose**.
Bradosol. Antiseptic for mouth and throat infections: see **Domiphen**.
Brasivol. Topical abrasive/cleansing paste for acne: see **Aluminium oxide**.
Bravit. Vitamin mixture: see **Aneurine, Nicotinic Acid, Pyridoxine, Riboflavine, Vitamin C**.
Breoprin. Sustained-release analgesic: see **Acetylsalicylic acid**.
Bretylate. Antidysrhythmic: see **Bretylium**.
Brevidil (d). Muscle relaxant used during anaesthesia: see **Suxamethonium**.
Brevinor. Oral contraceptive: see **Ethinyloestradiol, Norethisterone**.
Bricanyl. Sympathomimetic bronchodilator: see **Terbutaline**.
Bricanyl expectorant. Bronchodilator/expectorant. As Bricanyl plus **Guaiphenesin**.
Brietal Sodium. Short-acting barbiturate for short-duration anaesthesia: see **Methohexitone**.
Brinaldix K. Diuretic: see **Clopamide, Potassium chloride**.
Britcin. Antibiotic: see **Ampicillin**.
Brocadopa. Antiparkinsonian: see **Levodopa**.
Brocadopa Temtabs. Sustained-release formulation of Brocadopa.
Broflex. Antiparkinsonian/anticholinergic: see **Benzhexol**.
Brolene ophthalmic preps. Anti-infective drops/ointment for use in the eye: see **Propamidine**.
Bronchilator. Aerosol bronchodilator: see **Isoetharine, Phenylephrine**.
Bronchodil. Sympathetic bronchodilator: see **Reproterol**.
Brontisol (d). Aerosol bronchodilator: see **Deptropine, Isoprenaline**.
Brovon inhalant. Aerosol bronchodilator: see **Adrenaline, Atropine methonitrate, Papaverine**.
Broxil. Antibiotic: see **Phenethicillin**.
Brufen. Non-steroid anti-inflammatory/analgesic: see **Ibuprofen**.
Brulidine. Topical anti-infective for burns, wounds: see **Dibromopropamidine**.
Burinex. Diuretic: see **Bumetanide**.
Burinex K. As Burinex plus **Potassium chloride** supplement.
Buscopan. Anticholinergic/antispasmodic for gastro-intestinal or uterine spasm: see **Hyoscine butylbromide**.
Butacote. Non-steroid anti-inflammatory/analgesic: see **Phenylbutazone**. Enteric-coated to reduce gastric irritation.

Butazolidin. Non-steroid anti-inflammatory/analgesic: see **Phenylbutazone**.
Butazone. Non-steroid anti-inflammatory/analgesic: see **Phenylbutazone**.

C

Cafadol. Analgesic/antipyretic: see **Caffeine, Paracetamol**.
Cafergot. Vasoconstrictor for migraine: see **Caffeine, Ergotamine**.
Calaband. Impregnated bandage for dressing skin wounds and ulcers: see **Boric acid, Calamine, Castor oil, Glycerin, Modified starch, Zinc oxide**.
Caladryl. Cream or lotion for skin irritation (e.g., sunburn, insect bites): see **Calamine, Diphenhydramine**.
Calcimax. Calcium/vitamin supplements for calcium deficiencies: see **Aneurine, Hydroxocobalamin, Nicotinic acid, Pantothenic acid, Pyridoxine, Riboflavine, Vitamin C**.
Calciparine. Anticoagulant: see **Heparin**.
Calcisorb. For prevention of hypercalcuria and renal stones: see **Sodium cellulose phosphate**.
Calcitare. Hormone: see **Calcitonin**.
Calcium heparin. Anticoagulant: see **Heparin**.
Calcium leucovorin. Antagonizes antifolate cytotoxic drugs: see **Folinic acid**.
Calcium Resonium. Ion exchange resin: see **Calcium polystyrene sulphonate**.
Calcium-Sandoz. Calcium supplement for deficiency (e.g., tetany).
Calcuparine. Anticoagulant in pre-filled syringes for subcutaneous injection: see **Heparin**.
Callusolve. Topical treatment for warts: see **Benzalkonium**.
Calmurid. Keratolytic cream for removal of dry, scaly skin: see **Urea**.
Calmurid HC. Corticosteroid cream for eczema: see **Hydrocortisone, Urea**.
Calogen (b). Contains arachis oil, a source of high energy for use in renal failure.
Calonutrin (b). Mono-, di- and polysaccharide mixture free from lactose and sucrose.
Caloreen (b). Protein-free, high-calorie powder for use when low-protein diet is needed (e.g., kidney failure).
Calpol. Analgesic elixir: see **Paracetamol**.
Calsynar. Hormone: see **Calcitonin**.
Calthor. Antibiotic: see **Ciclacillin**.
C.A.M. Bronchodilator elixir for children: see **Butethamate, Ephedrine**.
Camcolit. Antidepressant for manic depressive psychosis: see **Lithium salts**.
Camoquin. Antimalarial: see **Amodiaquine**.
Canesten. Antifungal: see **Clotrimazole**.

Canesten HC. Topical anti-infective/corticosteroid. As **Canestan plus Hydrocortisone**.
Cantil. Anticholinergic for abdominal colic and diarrhoea: see **Mepenzolate**.
Capastat. Anti-tuberculous antibiotic: see **Capreomycin**.
Capitol (b). Shampoo for scaly scalp conditions: see **Benzalkonium**.
Caplenal. For gout: see **Allopurinol**.
Capoten. Antihypertensive: see **Captopril**.
Caprin. Slow-release analgesic: see **Acetylsalicylic acid**.
Carbellon. Antacid/sedative: see **Belladonna extract, Charcoal, Magnesium hydroxide**.
Carbo-Cort. Corticosteroid cream for eczema and other skin rashes: see **Coal tar, Hydrocortisone**.
Carbo-Dome. Topical treatment for psoriasis: see **Coal tar**.
Carbomix. Oral adsorbant for treatment of acute poisoning and drug overdose: see **Activated charcoal**.
Cardiacap. Antianginal: see **Pentaerythritol tetranitrate**.
Carisoma. Muscle relaxant: see **Carisoprodol**.
Carisoma compound. As Carisoma plus analgesic: see **Carisoprodol, Paracetamol**.
Carobel. Carob seed flour for thickening feeds in the treatment of vomiting.
Carylderm. Insecticide lotion shampoo for treatment of lice: see **Carbaryl**.
Cascara evacuant. Purgative: see **Cascara**.
Casilan (b). High-protein, low-salt food for hypoproteinaemia.
Catapres. Antihypertensive: see **Clonidine**.
Caved-S. For peptic ulcers: see **Aluminium hydroxide, Bismuth salts, Deglycyrrhizinised liquorice, Frangula, Magnesium carbonate, Sodium bicarbonate**.
CCNU. Cytotoxic: see **Lomustine**.
Ceanel (b). Shampoo for psoriasis: see **Cetrimide**.
Ce-Cobalin. Vitamins: see **Cyanocobalamin, Vitamin C**.
Cedilanid. For heart failure: see **Lanatoside C**.
Cedocard. Antianginal: see **Sorbide nitrate**.
Ceduran. Urinary anti-infective: see **Deglycyrrhizinised liquorice, Nitrofurantoin**.
Cefizox. Antibiotic: see **Ceftizoxime**.
Celbenin. Antibiotic: see **Methicillin**.
Celevac. Purgative: see **Methylcellulose**.
Cellucon. Purgative: see **Methylcellulose**.
Cendevax (d). **Rubella vaccine**.
Centrax. Anxiolytic: see **Prazepam**.
Centyl. Diuretic: see **Bendrofluazide**.
Centyl-K. Diuretic: see **Bendrofluazide, Potassium chloride**.
Ceporex. Antibiotic: see **Cephalexin**.
Ceporin (d). Antibiotic: see **Cephaloridine**.
Cerumol. Drops for removal of ear wax: see **Chlorbutol, Paradichlorobenzene, Turpentine oil**.

Cervagem. Pessary for use prior to surgical termination of pregnancy: see **Gemeprost**.
Cesamet. Anti-emetic: see **Nabilone**.
Cetavlex. Topical anti-infective for minor abrasions: see **Cetrimide**.
Cetavlon PC (b). Shampoo for seborrhoea: see **Cetrimide**.
Cetiprin. Anticholinergic used for relief of postoperative bladder pain and urinary frequency: see **Emepronium**.
Cetriclens. Antiseptic solution: see **Cetrimide, Chlorhexidine**.
Chemocycline. Antibiotic: see **Oxytetracycline**.
Chemotrim. Antibacterial: see **Co-trimoxazole**.
Chendol. Bile acid for dissolution of cholesterol gall stones: see **Cheno-deoxycholic acid**.
Chenocedon. Used to dissolve cholesterol gall stones: see **Cheno-deoxycholic acid**.
Chenofalk. Bile acid for dissolution of cholesterol gall stones: see **Cheno-deoxycholic acid**.
Chloractil. Major tranquillizer: see **Chlorpromazine**.
Chloraseptic. Lozenges, gargle or spray for sore throat: see **Phenol**.
Chlorasol. Solution for cleansing and desloughing of skin ulcers: see **Sodium hypochlorite**.
Chloromycetin. Anti-infective: see **Chloramphenicol**.
Chloromycetin hydrocortisone. Anti-infective/corticosteroid drops for infection/inflammation of eyes: see **Chloramphenicol, Hydrocortisone**.
Chocovite. For calcium deficiency: see **Calcium gluconate, Vitamin D**.
Choledyl. Bronchodilator: see **Choline theophyllinate**.
Choloxin. Lowers plasma cholesterol levels: see **Dextrothyroxine sodium**.
Chymar. Enzyme injection for post-traumatic tissue reactions: see **Chymotrypsin**.
Chymar-Zon. Enzyme extract used to aid extraction of the lens from the eye in cataract surgery: see **Chymotrypsin**.
Chymocyclar. Antibiotic plus enzymes: see **Tetracycline, Pancreatic enzymes**.
Chymoral. Oral enzyme preparation for post-traumatic tissue reactions: see **Pancreatic enzymes**.
Cicatrin. Topical anti-infective: see **Bacitracin, Neomycin**.
Cidomycin. Antibiotic for injection or topical use: see **Gentamicin**.
Cinobac. Antibacterial: see **Cinoxacin**.
Citanest. Local anaesthetic for minor surgery: see **Prilocaine**.
Citanest with Octapressin. As Citanest plus vasoconstrictor to prolong action: see **Felypressin**.
Claforan. Antibiotic: see **Cefotaxime**.
Clairvan. Respiratory stimulant: see **Ethamivan**.
Claradin. Effervescent analgesic: see **Acetylsalicylic acid**.
Clinifeed (b). Liquid feeds for enteral absorption. Given via naso-gastric tube or enterostomy as treatment or prevention of malnourishment (e.g., postoperatively).
Clinium. Antianginal: see **Lidoflazine**.
Clinitar. Cream and shampoo for psoriasis and eczema: see **Coal tar**.

Clinoril. Non-steroid anti-inflammatory/analgesic: see **Sulindac**.
Clomid. Sex hormone: see **Clomiphene**.
Clopixol. Major tranquillizer administered as long-acting injection: see **Clopenthixol**.
Cobadex. Corticosteroid ointment for dermatitis: see **Hydrocortisone**.
Cobalin-H. Vitamin B_{12} injection for treatment of B_{12}-deficient anaemia: see **Hydroxocobalamin**.
Co-Betaloc. Antihypertensive: see **Hydrochlorothiazide, Metoprolol**.
Cobutolin. Sympathomimetic bronchodilator: see **Salbutamol**.
Codelsol. Corticosteroid injection: see **Prednisolone**.
Codis. Soluble analgesic: see **Co-codaprin**.
Co-Ferol (d). Prophylactic treatment for anaemia of pregnancy: see **Ferrous fumarate, Folic acid**.
Cogentin. Anticholinergic/antiparkinsonian: see **Benztropine**.
Colestid. For reduction of high blood cholesterol levels: see **Colestipol**.
Colifoam. Corticosteroid in aerosol foam for topical treatment of inflammation of large bowel: see **Hydrocortisone**.
Colofac. Antispasmodic for abdominal colic: see **Mebeverine**.
Cologel. Purgative: see **Methylcellulose**.
Colomycin. Anti-infective: see **Polymyxin B**.
Colpermin. Used for intestinal colic: see **Pepperment oil**.
Coltapaste. Impregnated bandage: see **Coal tar, Zinc oxide**.
Colven. Purgative/antispasmodic for treatment of bowel dysfunction and abdominal pain (e.g., irritable bowel syndrome): see **Ispaghula mebeverine**.
Combantrin. For treatment of infections due to threadworm, roundworm, and trichostrongyliasis: see **Pyrantel**.
Combizym (d). For use in pancreatic deficiency: see **Pancreatic enzymes**.
Combizym Composition (d). For use in pancreatic deficiency: see **Bile salts, Pancreatic enzymes**.
Comminuted chicken meat (b). For use in carbohydrate and milk protein intolerance in infancy.
Comox. Antibacterial: see **Co-trimoxazole**.
Comploment. Sustained-release vitamin preparation for treatment of depression due to pyridoxine deficiency and the oral contraceptive: see **Pyridoxine**.
Concavit. Vitamin mixture: see **Aneurine, Cyanocobalamin, Pantothenic acid, Nicotinamide, Pyridoxine, Riboflavine, Vitamin A, Vitamin C**.
Concordin. Antidepressant: see **Protriptyline**.
Congesteze. Antihistamine/sympathomimetic for treatment of common cold: see **Azatadine, Pseudoephedrine**.
Conjuvac. Vaccine for desensitization against two common grasses: see **Allergen extract vaccine**.
Conotrane. Topical anti-infective: see **Hydrargaphen**.
Conova 30. Oral contraceptive: see **Ethinyloestradiol, Ethynodiol**.
Controvlar. For menstrual irregularities: see **Ethinyloestradiol, Norethisterone**.

Coparvax. Bacterial suspension (*Cornyebacterium parvum*), instilled into the pleural or peritoneal cavities to treat malignant effusions and ascites.
Copholco. Cough suppressant: see **Pholcodine**.
Cordarone X. Antidysrhythmic: see **Amiodarone**.
Cordilox. Antianginal/antihypertensive: see **Verapamil**.
Corgard. Antihypertensive: see **Nadolol**.
Corgaretic. Antihypertensive: see **Bendrofluazide, Nadolol**.
Corlan. Corticosteroid pellet for aphthous ulcers: see **Hydrocortisone**.
Coro-nitro. Oral spray for angina pectoris: see **Glyceryl trinitrate**.
Corsodyl. Topical treatment for gingivitis: see **Chlorhexidine**.
Cortacream. Impregnated bandage: see **Hydrocortisone**.
Cortelan. Corticosteroid: see **Cortisone**.
Cortenema. Corticosteroid enema for colitis: see **Hydrocortisone**.
Cortistab. Corticosteroid: see **Cortisone**.
Cortisyl. Corticosteroid: see **Cortisone**.
Cortucid. Corticosteroid eye drops: see **Hydrocortisone, Sulphacetamide**.
Cosalgesic (d). Analgesic: see **Co-proxamol**.
Cosmegen Lyovac. Cytotoxic: see **Actinomycin D**.
Cosuric. For gout: see **Allopurinol**.
Cosylan. Cough suppressant: see **Dextromethorphan**.
Cotazym. For use in pancreatic deficiency: see **Pancreatic enzymes**.
Cotrimox. Antibiotic: see **Co-trimoxazole**.
Covering Cream (b). Concealing cream: see **Titanium dioxide**.
Covermark (b). Concealing cream: see **Titanium dioxide**.
Cremalgex. Rubefacient: see **Glycol salicylate, Histamine, Methyl nicotinate**.
Cremalgin. Rubefacient: see **Glycol salicylate, Histamine, Methyl nicotinate**.
Cremathurm R. Rubefacient: see **Ethyl nicotinate, Histamine, Methyl salicylate**.
Creon. Used with food in pancreatic insufficiency: see **Pancreatic enzymes**.
Crescormon. Human growth hormone injection for treatment of short stature: see **Growth hormone, Somatotrophin**.
Crystapen. Antibiotic: see **Benzylpenicillin**.
Crystapen G (d). Antibiotic: see **Benzylpenicillin**.
Crystapen V. Antibiotic: see **Phenoxymethylpenicillin**.
Cuplex. Topical treatment for removal of warts, corns and callouses: see **Copper acetate, Lactic acid, Salicylic acid**.
Cyclimorph (c). Narcotic analgesic: see **Cyclizine, Morphine**.
Cyclobral. Peripheral vasodilator for peripheral vascular disease and impaired mental function due to cerebrovascular disease: see **Cyclandelate**.
Cyclogest. Suppository for treatment of premenstrual symptoms: see **Progesterone**.
Cyclo-Progynova. Sex hormones for menopausal symptoms: see **Norgestrel, Oestradiol**.
Cyclo-Prostin (d). Vasodilator, platelet aggregation inhibitor: see **Epoprostenol**.

Cycloserine. Antibiotic used in tuberculosis and in urinary tract infections: see **Cycloserine**.
Cyclospasmol. Peripheral vasodilator: see **Cyclandelate**.
Cyklokapron. Anti-fibrinolytic: see **Tranexamic acid**.
Cyprostat. Sex hormone for treatment of prostatic carcinoma: see **Cyproterone**.
Cytacon. For vitamin B_{12} deficiency: see **Cyanocobalamin**.
Cytamen. For vitamin B_{12}-deficient anaemias: see **Cyanocobalamin**.
Cyteal. Antiseptic skin cleanser: see **Chlorhexidine, Chlorocresol, Hexamidine** (isethionate).
Cytosar. Cytotoxic: see **Cytarabine**.

D

Dactil. Gut antispasmodic: see **Piperidolate**.
Dactinomycin. See **Actinomycin D**.
Daktacort. Topical anti-infective/corticosteroid: see **Hydrocortisone, Miconazole**.
Daktarin. Topical antifungal for skin and nails: see **Miconazole**.
Dalacin C. Antibiotic: see **Clindamycin**.
Dalivit. Multivitamin preparation: see **Ascorbic acid, Calcium pentothenate, Nicotinamide, Pyridoxine, Riboflavine, Thiamine, Vitamin A, Vitamin D**.
Dalmane. Hypnotic: see **Flurazepam**.
Daneral-SA. Anti-allergic: see **Pheniramine**.
Danol. Semisynthetic steroid used in endometriosis: see **Danazol**.
Dantrium. Muscle relaxant: see **Dantrolene**.
Daonil. Oral hypoglycaemic: see **Glibenclamide**.
Daranide. Diuretic used in states of respiratory acidosis: see **Dichlorphenamide**.
Daraprim. Antimalarial: see **Pyrimethamine**.
Dartalan (d). Tranquillizer/anti-emetic: see **Thiopropazate**.
Davenol. Decongestant/cough suppressant: see **Carbinoxamine, Ephedrine, Pholcodine**.
Dayovite. Source of oral vitamins B and C.
DDAVP. Synthetic antidiuretic hormone: see **Desmopressin**.
Deanase. Enzyme injection for local inflammatory disorders: see **Deoxyribonuclease**.
Deanase D.C. Oral enzyme for inflammatory disorders: see **Chymotrypsin**.
Debendox (d). Antiemetic: see **Dicyclomine, Doxylamine, Pyridoxine**.
Debrisan. Powder used to aid healing of wounds: see **Dextranomer**.
Debroxide. Topical treatment for acne: see **Benzoyl peroxide**.
Decadron. Corticosteroid: see **Dexamethasone**.
Deca-Durabolin. Anabolic steroid: see **Nandrolone**.

Decaserpyl. Antihypertensive: see **Methoserpidine**.
Decaserpyl plus. Antihypertensive: see **Benzthiazide, Methoserpidine**.
Declinax. Antihypertensive: see **Debrisoquine**.
Decortisyl. Corticosteroid: see **Prednisone**.
Defencin. Cerebral and peripheral vasodilator: see **Isoxsuprine**.
Delfen. Spermicidal contraceptive: see **Nonoxynol**.
Delimon. Analgesic: see **Morazone, Paracetamol**.
Deltacortril. Corticosteroid tablets or injection: see **Prednisolone**.
Deltacortril-enteric. Corticosteroid. Enteric coating said to reduce gastric irritation: see **Prednisolone**.
Deltalone. Corticosteroid: see **Prednisolone**.
Delta-Phoricol. Corticosteroid: see **Prednisolone**.
Deltastab. Corticosteroid tablets or injection: see **Prednisolone**.
Demser. Antihypertensive: see **Metirosine**.
De-Nol. For treatment of peptic ulcer: see **Tri-potassium dicitrato bismuthate**.
De-Noltab. Antacid, tablet formulation of De-Nol.
Depixol. Major tranquillizer: see **Flupenthixol**.
Depocillin. Antibiotic: see **Procaine penicillin**.
Depo-Medrone. Corticosteroid for intra-articular/intramuscular injection: see **Methylprednisolone**.
Depo-Provera. Progestogen, depo-injection used in threatened abortion, endometriosis: see **Medroxyprogesterone**.
Depostat. Progestogen, depo-injection for benign prostatic hypertrophy: see **Gestronol**.
Dequacaine. Local anaesthetic lozenges: see **Benzocaine, Dequalinium**.
Dequadin. Antiseptic throat lozenges: see **Dequalinium**.
Derbac liquid. Topical anaesthetic cream: see **Cinchocaine**.
Dermalex. Soothing antiseptic lotion for prevention of bed sores or urine rash: see **Allantoin, Hexachlorophane, Squalane**.
Dermonistat. Topical antifungal: see **Miconazole**.
Dermovate. Topical steroid treatments: see **Clobetasol**.
Dermovate-NN. Topical corticosteroid/anti-infective: see **Clobetasol, Neomycin, Nystatin**.
Deseril. Antiserotoninergic: see **Methysergide**.
Desferal. Chelating agent: see **Desferrioxamine**.
Destolit. Bile acid for dissolution of cholesterol gall stones: see **Ursodeoxycholic acid**.
Deteclo. Antibiotic: see **Chlortetracycline, Demeclocycline, Tetracycline**.
Dettol. Topical antiseptic: see **Chloroxylenol**.
Dexa-Rhinaspray. Nasal spray for allergic or chronic rhinitis: see **Dexamethasone, Neomycin, Tramazoline**.
Dexedrine (c). CNS stimulant: see **Dexamphetamine**.
Dextraven 110/150. Plasma expanders: see **Dextrans**.
Dextrogesic (d). Analgesic: see **Co-proxamol**.
Dextrolyte. Oral electrolyte solution: see **Glucose, Potassium chloride, Sodium lactate**.
DF 118. Analgesic: see **Dihydrocodeine**. (c) injection but not tablets.

Diabinese. Oral hypoglycaemic: see **Chlorpropamide**.
Diamicron. Oral hypoglycaemic: see **Gliclazide**.
Diamox. Diuretic: see **Acetazolamide**.
Diane. Hormone treatment for acne and hirsutism: see **Cyproterone, Ethinyloestradiol**.
Diarrest. Antidiarrhoeal: see **Codeine, Dicyclomine, Potassium chloride, Sodium chloride, Sodium citrate**.
Diatensec. Diuretic: see **Spironolactone**.
Dia-Tuss. Cough linctus: see **Pholcodeine**.
Diazemuls. Anxiolytic for injection, formulated as an oil-in-water emulsion. May be used in patients where injection of an aqueous solution causes thrombophlebitis or pain during injection: see **Diazepam**.
Dibenyline. Alpha-adrenoceptor blocker: see **Phenoxybenzamine**.
Diconal (c). Analgesic: see **Dipipanone**.
Dicynene. Haemostatic: see **Ethamsylate**.
Didronel. Used in Paget's disease: see **Etidronate disodium**.
Difflam. Topical, non-steroid anti-inflammatory/analgesic cream: see **Benzydamine**.
Digitaline Nativelle. Cardiac glycoside: see **Digitoxin**.
Dihydergot. For migraine: see **Dihydroergotamine**.
Dijex. Antacid: see **Aluminium hydroxide, Magnesium carbonate**.
Dimelor. Oral hypoglycaemic: see **Acetohexamide**.
Dimotane. Antihistamine: see **Brompheniramine**.
Dimotane Expectorant. Expectorant cough mixture: see **Brompheniramine, Guaiphenesin, Phenylephrine, Phenylpropanolamine**.
Dimotane Expectorant DC (c). Cough linctus/expectorant. Similar to Dimotane Expectorant plus **Dihydrocodeine**.
Dimotane LA. Sustained-release formulation of Dimotane.
Dimotane with codeine. Cough linctus similar to Dimotane Expectorant plus **Codeine**.
Dimotapp. Antihistamine/decongestant for symptomatic treatment of common cold. Available as sustained-release and elixir formulations: see **Brompheniramine, Phenylephrine, Phenylpropanolamine**.
Dimotapp P. Analgesic/decongestant: see **Brompheniramine, Paracetamol, Phenylephrine, Phenylpropanolamine**.
Dimyril. Cough suppressant: see **Isoaminile citrate**.
Dindevan. Anticoagulant: see **Phenindione**.
Dioctyl ear capsules. Oil for removal of ear wax: see **Dioctyl sodium sulphosuccinate**.
Dioctyl-Medo. Purgative: see **Dioctyl sodium sulphosuccinate**.
Dioderm. Corticosteroid cream for inflammatory and allergic skin conditions: see **Hydrocortisone**.
Dioralyte. Electrolytes and dextrose supplied in a powder for reconstitution into a solution. Used orally to correct fluid and electrolyte balance (e.g., due to diarrhoea and vomiting).
Diovol. Antacid: see **Aluminium hydroxide, Dimethicone, Magnesium hydroxide**.

Diprobase. Cream or ointment for topical application to dry skin: see **Cetomacrogol, Cetostearyl alcohol, Liquid paraffin, Soft paraffin**.
Diprosalic. Ointment and lotion for dermatitis: see **Betamethasone, Salicylic acid**.
Diprosone. Topical corticosteroid: see **Betamethasone**.
Dirythmin-SA. Sustained-release antidysrhythmic: see **Disopyramide**.
Disadine. Dry powder spray for skin disinfection: see **Povidone-iodine**.
Disalcid. Analgesic: see **Salsalate**.
Disipal. Anticholinergic/antiparkinsonian: see **Orphenadrine**.
Di-Sipidin. Hormone extract: see **Posterior pituitary extract**.
Distaclor. Antibiotic: see **Cefaclor**.
Distalgesic. Analgesic: see **Dextropropoxyphene, Paracetamol**.
Distamine. Chelating agent used in rheumatoid arthritis: see **Penicillamine**.
Distaquaine V-K. Antibiotic: see **Phenoxymethylpenicillin**.
Dithrocream. Cream for treatment of quiescent psoriasis: see **Dithranol**.
Dithrolan. Topical treatment of quiescent psoriasis: see **Dithranol, Salicyclic acid**.
Diumide K. Diuretic with sustained-release potassium: see **Frusemide, Potassium chloride**.
Diuresal. Diuretic: see **Frusemide**.
Diurexan. Diuretic/antihypertensive: see **Xipamide**.
Dixarit. Migraine prophylactic: see **Clonidine**.
Dobutrex. Infusion for treatment of severe heart failure: see **Dobutamine**.
Dolasan. Analgesic: see **Acetylsalicylic acid, Dextropropoxyphene**.
Dolmatil. Antipsychotic: see **Sulpiride**.
Dolobid. Analgesic: see **Diflunisal**.
Doloxene. Analgesic: see **Dextropropoxyphene**.
Doloxene compound. Analgesic: see **Acetylsalicylic acid, Caffeine, Dextropropoxyphene**.
Dome-Acne. Topical treatment for acne: see **Resorcinol, Salicylic acid, Sulphur**.
Dome-Cort cream. Corticosteroid cream: see **Hydrocortisone**.
Domical. Antidepressant: see **Amitriptyline**.
Dopamet. Antihypertensive: see **Methyldopa**.
Dopram. Respiratory stimulant: see **Doxopram**.
Dorbanex. Purgative: see **Co-danthramer**.
Dormonoct. Hypnotic: see **Loprazolam**.
Double Check. Spermicidal contraceptive: see **Nonoxynol**.
Doxatet. Antibiotic: see **Doxycycline**.
Doxylar. Antibiotic: see **Doxycycline**.
Dozic. Tranquillizer: see **Haloperidol**.
Dozine. Antipsychotic: see **Chlorpromazine**.
Dramamine. Anti-emetic: see **Dimenhydrinate**.
Drapolene. Topical anti-infective: see **Benzalkonium**.
Driclor. Topical antiperspirant for hyperhidrosis: see **Aluminium chloride**.
Droleptan. Premedicant, major tranquillizer: see **Droperidol**.

Dromoran (c). Narcotic analgesic: see **Levorphanol**.
Droxalin. Antacid: see **Alexitol sodium, Magnesium trisilicate**.
Dryptal. Diuretic: see **Frusemide**.
DTIC. Cytotoxic: see **Dacarbazine**.
Dubam. Rubefacient, pain-relieving spray: see **Ethyl salicylate, Glycol salicylate, Methyl nicotinate, Methyl salicylate**.
Dulcodos. Laxative: see **Bisacodyl, Dioctyl sodium sulphosuccinate**.
Dulcolax. Laxative: see **Bisacodyl**.
Duo-Autohaler. Aerosol bronchodilator: see **Isoprenaline, Phenylephrine**.
Duofilm. Topical treatment for warts: see **Lactic acid, Salicylic acid**.
Duogastrone. Position release preparation for duodenal ulcer: see **Carbenoxolone**.
Duovent. Bronchodilator for inhalation: see **Fenoterol, Ipratropium**.
Duphalac. Purgative: see **Lactulose**.
Duphaston. For dysmenorrhoea and endometriosis: see **Dydrogesterone**.
Durabolin. Anabolic steroid: see **Nandrolone**.
Duracreme. Spermicidal contraceptive: see **Nonoxynol**.
Duragel. Spermicidal jelly used for contraception: see **Nonoxynol**.
Duromine (c). Anti-obesity: see **Phentermine**.
Duromorph (c). Narcotic analgesic: see **Morphine**.
Durophet (c). Anti-obesity: see **Amphetamine**.
Duvadilan. Peripheral vasodilator: see **Isoxsuprine**.
Dyazide. Diuretic combination: see **Hydrochlorothiazide, Triamterene**.
Dynese. Antacid: see **Magaldrate**.
Dytac. Diuretic: see **Triamterene**.
Dytide. Diuretic combination: see **Benzthiazide, Triamterene**.

E

E 45 cream. Skin-protective, paraffin-based cream.
Ebufac. Non-steroid anti-inflammatory/analgesic: see **Ibuprofen**.
Econacort. Topical treatment of fungal/bacterial skin infections: see **Econazole, Hydrocortisone**.
Econocil V-K. Antibiotic: see **Phenoxymethylpenicillin**.
Economycin. Antibiotic: see **Tetracycline**.
Econosone. Corticosteroid: see **Prednisone**.
Ecostatin. Antifungal for topical use: see **Econazole**.
Eczederm. Soothing cream for skin application: see **Calamine**.
Edecrin. Diuretic: see **Ethacrynic acid**.
Efcortelan. Topical corticosteroid: see **Hydrocortisone**.
Efcortesol inj. Intravenous corticosteroid: see **Hydrocortisone**.
Effercitrate. Effervescent formulation for treatment of cystitis: see **Potassium citrate**.
Effico. 'Tonic': see **Aneurine, Caffeine, Nicotinamide, Strychnine**.
Efudix. Cytotoxic: see **Fluorouracil**.

Elantan. Antianginal: see **Isosorbide mononitrate**.
Elavil. Antidepressant: see **Amitriptyline**.
Eldepryl. Used with **Levodopa** in treatment of Parkinson's disease: see **Selegiline**.
Eldisine. Cytotoxic: see **Vindesine**.
Electrosol. Soluble tablets for electrolyte depletion: see **Potassium chloride, Sodium bicarbonate, Sodium chloride**.
Elemental 028 (b). Dietary substitute for use in malabsorption states and undernourished patients.
Eltroxin. Thyroid hormone: see **Thyroxine**.
Eludril. Antiseptic solution/aerosol for oral infections: see **Amethocaine, Chlorhexidine**.
Emeside. Anticonvulsant: see **Ethosuximide**.
Emetrol. Solution for treatment of nausea and vomiting including morning sickness in pregnancy, motion sickness and regurgitation in infants: see **Dextrose, Laevulose, Phosphoric acid**.
Emko. Spermicidal contraceptive: see **Benzethonium, Nonoxynol**.
Emla. Local anaesthetic cream for topical application in children to alleviate the pain of venepuncture: see **Lignocaine, Prilocaine**.
Emtexate. Cytotoxic: see **Methotrexate**.
Emulsiderm. Soothing, protective skin cream: see **Benzalkonium chloride, Liquid paraffin**.
EN-De-KAY. For prevention of dental caries: see **Sodium fluoride**.
Endoxana. Cytotoxic: see **Cyclophosphamide**.
Enduron. Diuretic: see **Methylclothiazide**.
Enrich (b). Liquid feed for enteral absorption.
Ensure. Liquid source of calories for oral nutrition in debilitating conditions.
Entamizole. Amoebicide: see **Diloxanide**.
Enteromide. Antibacterial/antidiarrhoeal: see **Calcium sulphaloxate**.
Epanutin. Anticonvulsant: see **Phenytoin**.
Ephynal. Tocopheryl: see **Vitamin E**.
Epifoam. Corticosteroid/local anaesthetic aerosol foam for topical use (e.g., in peri-anal trauma): see **Hydrocortisone, Pramoxine**.
Epifrin. Eye drops for narrow-angle glaucoma: see **Adrenaline**.
Epilim. Anticonvulsant: see **Sodium valproate**.
Epodyl. Cytotoxic: see **Ethoglucid**.
Eppy. Eye drops for glaucoma: see **Adrenaline**.
Epsikapron. Haemostatic: see **Epsilon-aminocaproic acid**.
Equagesic. Anti-inflammatory/analgesic: see **Acetylsalicylic acid, Calcium carbonate, Ethoheptazine, Meprobamate**.
Equanil. Sedative/tranquillizer: see **Meprobamate**.
Equivert. Anti-emetic, antivertigo: see **Buclizine, Nicotinic acid**.
Eradacin. Antibacterial: see **Acrosoxacin**.
Ermysin. Antibiotic: see **Erythromycin**.
Ervevax. Vaccine for immunization against rubella (German measles): see **Rubella vaccine**.
Erycen. Antibiotic: see **Erythromycin**.

Erymax. Antibiotic: see **Erythromycin**.
Erythrocin. Antibiotic: see **Erythromycin**.
Erythrolar. Antibiotic: see **Erythromycin**.
Erythromid. Antibiotic: see **Erythromycin**.
Erythroped. Antibiotic: see **Erythromycin**.
Esbatal. Antihypertensive: see **Bethanidine**.
Esidrex. Diuretic: see **Hydrochlorothiazide**.
Esidrex-K. As Esidrex plus **Potassium chloride** supplement.
Eskamel. Cream for acne: see **Resorcinol, Sulphur**.
Eskornade. Anticholinergic/sympathomimetic/antihistamine mixture for symptomatic treatment of common cold: see **Diphenylpyraline, Isopropamide, Phenylpropanolamine**.
Esoderm (b). Shampoo for head lice: see **Dicophane, Gamma-benzene hexachloride**.
Estracyt. Cytotoxic for carcinoma of the prostate: see **Estramustine phosphate**.
Estradurin. Sex hormone for carcinoma of the prostate: see **Polyoestradiol**.
Estrovis. For suppression of lactation: see **Quinestrol**.
Ethrane. Inhalational anaesthetic: see **Enflurane**.
Eudemine. Antihypertensive/hyperglycaemic: see **Diazoxide**.
Euglucon. Oral hypoglycaemic: see **Glibenclamide**.
Eugynon 30 and 50. Oral contraceptives: see **Ethinyloestradiol, Norgestrel**.
Euhypnos. Hypnotic: see **Temazepam**.
Eumovate. Corticosteroid eye drops: cream or ointment for skin see **Clobetasone**.
Eumovate – N. As Eumovate plus **Neomycin**.
Eumydrin. Anticholinergic: see **Atropine methonitrate**.
Eurax. Topical antipruritic: see **Crotamiton**.
Eurax-hydrocortisone. As Eurax plus **Hydrocortisone**.
Evacalm. Anxiolytic: see **Diazepam**.
Evadyne. Antidepressant: see **Butriptyline**.
Exelderm. Topical antifungal for skin infections: see **Sulconazole**.
Exirel. Sympathomimetic bronchodilator: see **Pirbuterol**.
Exolan. Topical treatments for psoriasis: see **Dithranol**.
Expansyl Spansule (d). Slow-release bronchodilator: see **Diphenylpyraline, Ephedrine, Trifluoperazine**.
Expulin. Cough linctus: see **Chlorpheniramine, Ephedrine, Menthol, Pholcodine**.
Expurhin Paediatric Decongestant. Decongestant linctus: see **Chlorpheniramine, Ephedrine, Menthol**.
Exterol. Drops for removal of ear wax: see **Urea hydrogen peroxide**.
Extil compound linctus. Cough linctus: see **Carbinoxamine, Noscapine, Pseudoephedrine**.
Exyphen. Cough linctus: see **Brompheniramine, Guaiphenesin, Phenylephrine, Phenylpropanolamine**.

F

Fabahistin. Antihistamine: see **Mebhydroline**.

Fabrol. Mucolytic: see **Acetylcysteine**.

Fansidar. Antimalarial: see **Pyrimethamine**.

Farlutal. Sex hormone for treatment of hormone-dependent malignancies: see **Medroxyprogesterone acetate**.

Fasigyn. Antimicrobial: see **Tinidazole**.

FEAC. Slow-release haematinic with vitamins: see **Aneurine, Ferrous sulphate, Nicotinamide, Pyridoxine, Riboflavine, Vitamin C**.

Fe-Cap. Haematinic: see **Ferrous glycine sulphate**.

Fe-Cap C. As Fe-Cap plus **Vitamin C**.

Fe-Cap folic. As Fe-Cap plus **Folic acid**.

Fectrim. Antibacterial: see **Co-trimoxazole**.

Fefol Spansule. Slow-release haematinic: see **Ferrous sulphate, Folic acid**.

Fefol-Vit Spansule. As Fefol Spansule plus vitamins: see **Aneurine, Nicotinic acid, Pantothenic acid, Pyridoxine, Riboflavine**.

Fefol Z. Sustained-release haematinic: see **Ferrous sulphate, Folic acid, Zinc sulphate**.

Feldene. Non-steroid anti-inflammatory/analgesic: see **Piroxicam**.

Femerital. Analgesic for dysmenorrhoea: see **Ambucetamide, Paracetamol**.

Femulen. Oral contraceptive: see **Ethynodiol**.

Fenbid. Sustained-release non-steroid anti-inflammatory/analgesic: see **Ibuprofen**.

Fenopron. Non-steroid anti-inflammatory/analgesic: see **Fenoprofen**.

Fenostil retard. Antihistamine: see **Dimethindene**.

Fentazin. Tranquillizer/anti-emetic: see **Perphenazine**.

Feospan Spansule. Slow-release haematinic: see **Ferrous sulphate**.

Feospan Z. Sustained-release haematinic: see **Ferrous sulphate, Zinc sulphate**.

Ferfolic M. Haematinic for prevention of anaemia of pregnancy: see **Ferrous gluconate, Folic acid, Vitamin C**.

Ferfolic SV (d). Haematinic for folic acid-deficient anaemias. Similar contents to Ferfolic M but higher **Folic acid** content.

Fergluvite (d). Haematinic/vitamins. Similar to Ferfolic but no **Folic acid**.

Fergon. Haematinic: see **Ferrous gluconate**.

Ferrocap. Slow-release haematinic: see **Aneurine, Ferrous fumarate**.

Ferrocap F 350. Slow-release haematinic: see **Ferrous fumarate, Folic acid**.

Ferrocontin continus. Sustained-release haematinic: see **Ferrous glycine sulphate**.

Ferrocontin Folic Continus. Sustained-release haematinic: see **Ferrous glycine sulphate, Folic acid**.

Ferrograd C. Slow-release haematinic/vitamin: see **Ferrous sulphate, Vitamin C**.

Ferrograd Folic. Slow-release haematinic: see **Ferrous sulphate, Folic acid**.

Ferro-Gradumet. Slow-release haematinic: see **Ferrous sulphate**.
Ferromyn. Haematinic: see **Ferrous succinate**.
Ferromyn B. Haematinic/vitamins: see **Aneurine, Ferrous succinate, Nicotinic acid, Riboflavine**.
Ferromyn S. Haematinic: see **Ferrous succinate, Folic acid, Succinic acid**.
Fersaday. Slow-release haematinic: see **Ferrous fumarate**.
Fersamal. Haematinic: see **Ferrous fumarate**.
Fertiral. Hormone: see **Gonadorelin**.
Fesovit Spansule. Slow-release haematinic/vitamins: see **Aneurine, Ferrous sulphate, Nicotinic acid, Panthothenic acid, Pyridoxine, Riboflavine, Vitamin C**.
Fesovit Z. Sustained-release haematinic plus vitamins: see **Ferrous sulphate, Ascorbic acid, Nicotinamide, Pyridoxine, Riboflavine, Thiamine, Zinc sulphate**.
Finalgon. Rubefacient: see **Butoxyethyl nicotinate, Nonylic acid**.
Flagyl. Antibacterial: see **Metronidazole**.
Flagyl Compak. Anti-infective: see **Metronidazole, Nystatin**.
Flagyl-S. Antibacterial suspension: see **Benzoylmetroinidazole**.
Flamazine. Anti-infective cream for burns: see **Silver sulphadiazine**.
Flar. Compound vitamins for prevention of gastric side effects due to antibiotics: see **Aneurine, Cyanocobalamin, Folic acid, Inositol nicotinate, Liver extracts, Nicotinamide, Pantothenic acid, Pyroxidine, Riboflavine**.
Flavelix (d). Decongestant: see **Ammonium chloride, Ephedrine, Mepyramine, Sodium citrate**.
Flaxedil. Muscle relaxant: see **Gallamine**.
Fletcher's Enemette. Laxative enema: see **Docusate sodium**.
Fletcher's Phosphate Enema. Purgative: see **Sodium acid phosphate, Sodium phosphate**.
Flexical (b). High-calorie food with vitamins and minerals.
Florinef. Adrenocorticosteroid: see **Fludrocortisone**.
Floxapen. Antibiotic: see **Flucloxacillin**.
Fluanxol. Antidepressant/tranquillizer: see **Flupenthixol**.
Fluor-a-Day Lac. For prevention of dental caries: see **Sodium fluoride**.
Fluorigard. For prevention of dental caries: see **Sodium fluoride**.
Fluothane. Anaesthetic gas: see **Halothane**.
Fluvirin. Influenza vaccine for immunization.
FML. Corticosteroid eye drops: see **Fluorometholone**.
FML-Neo. Topical corticosteroid/antibiotic: see **Fluoromethalone, Neomycin**.
Folex-350. Haematinic: see **Ferrous fumarate, Folic acid**.
Folicin. Haematinic for prevention of anaemia in pregnancy: see **Ferrous sulphate, Folic acid, Copper sulphate, Manganese sulphate**.
Forane. General anaesthetic: see **Isoflurane**.
Forceval. Multivitamin and mineral supplement.
Forceval protein (b). Protein, vitamin and mineral supplements for low-sodium/low-fat diets.
Fortagesic. Analgesic: see **Paracetamol, Pentazocine**.
Fortral. Analgesic: see **Pentazocine**.

Fortum. Antibiotic: see **Ceftazidime**.
Fortunan. Tranquillizer: see **Haloperidol**.
Fosfor. 'Tonic': see **Phosphorylcolamine**.
Framycort. Topical anti-infective/corticosteroid: see **Framycetin/ Hydrocortisone**.
Framygen cream. Topical anti-infective for ear, eye, skin: see **Framycetin**.
Franol (c). Bronchodilator/sedative: see **Ephedrine, Phenobarbitone, Theophylline**.
Franol expectorant (c). Bronchodilator/sedative/expectorant. As Franol plus **Guaiphenesin**.
Franol plus (c). As Franol plus **Thenyldiamine**.
Fre Amine. Amino acids and electrolytes for intravenous nutrition.
Frisium. Anxiolytic/anticonvulsant: see **Clobazam**.
Froben. Non-steroid anti-inflammatory analgesic: see **Flurbiprofen**.
Frumil. Diuretic combination: see **Amiloride, Frusemide**.
Frusene. Diuretic combination: see **Frusemide, Triamterene**.
Frusetic. Diuretic: see **Frusemide**.
Frusid. Diuretic: see **Frusemide**.
Fucibet. Topical cream for skin infections: see **Betamethasone, Fusidic acid**.
Fucidin. Antibiotic: see **Fusidic acid**.
Fucidin H oint. and gel. Topical anti-infective/corticosteroid: see **Fusidic acid, Hydrocortisone**.
Fucidin Intertulle. Antibiotic gauze dressing: see **Fusidic acid**.
Fulcin 125 and 500. Antifungal: see **Griseofulvin**.
Fungilin. Antifungal: see **Amphotericin B**.
Fungizone intravenous. Antifungal injection: see **Amphotericin B**.
Furacin. Anti-infective: see **Nitrofurazone**.
Furadantin. Urinary anti-infective: see **Nitrofurantoin**.
Furamide. Anti-amoebic: see **Diloxanide**.
Furan (d). Urinary anti-infective: see **Nitrofurantoin**.
Fybogel. Laxative for diverticular disease, constipation: see **Ispaghula husk**.
Fybranta. Laxative for diverticular disease, constipation: see **Bran**.

G

Galactomin Preps (b). Low-lactose dietary supplement.
Galcodine. Cough suppressant: see **Codeine**.
Galenomycin. Antibiotic: see **Oxytetracycline**.
Galfer and Galfer F.A. For iron and folic acid-deficiency anaemias: see **Ferrous fumarate, Folic acid**.
Galfer-Vit. Compound iron and vitamin preparation.
Galphol. Cough suppressant: see **Pholcodine**.

Galpseud. Decongestant for relief of nasal, sinus, and upper respiratory tract congestion: see **Pseudoephedrine**.
Gamanil. Antidepressant: see **Lofepramine**.
Gammabulin. Concentrate of antibodies for prophylaxis against hepatitis A, measles and rubella: see **Immunoglobulin G**.
Gammonativ. Injection of **Immunoglobulin**.
Ganda. Eye drops for glaucoma: see **Guanethidine**.
Gantrisin. Antibacterial: see **Sulphafurazole**.
Garamycin. Antibiotic: see **Gentamicin**.
Gardenal sodium (c). Anticonvulsant: see **Phenobarbitone**.
Gastrils. Antacid: see **Aluminium hydroxide, Magnesium carbonate**.
Gastrocote. Antacid: see **Alginic acid, Aluminium hydroxide, Magnesium trisilicate, Sodium bicarbonate**.
Gastrovite. For iron and calcium deficiency: see **Calciferol, Calcium gluconate, Ferrous sulphate, Vitamin C**.
Gastrozepin. Selective anticholinergic for treatment of peptic ulcers: see **Pirenzepine**.
Gaviscon. Antacid: see **Alginic Acid, Aluminium hydroxide, Magnesium trisilicate, Sodium bicarbonate**.
Gelcotar. Topical treatment for psoriasis: see **Coal tar**.
Gelofusine. Plasma expander: see **Gelatin, Sodium chloride**.
Gelusil. Antacid: see **Aluminium hydroxide, Magnesium trisilicate**.
Genexol. Spermicidal pessary: see **Spermicides**.
Genisol (b). Topical treatment for scalp seborrhoeic dermatitis: see **Coal tar**.
Genticin. Antibiotic for topical and parenteral use: see **Gentamicin**.
Gentisone HC. Anti-inflammatory/anti-infective drops for outer ear: see **Gentamicin, Hydrocortisone**.
Gentran. Plasma expander: see **Dextrans, Sodium chloride**.
Gentran 40/Gentran 70. Plasma expanders: see **Dextrans**.
Gestanin. For recurrent abortion: see **Allyloestrenol**.
Gevral. Multivitamins and minerals for general deficiencies.
Givitol. Compound iron and vitamin preparation.
Glibenese. Oral hypoglycaemic: see **Glipizide**.
Glucophage. Oral hypoglycaemic: see **Metformin**.
Glucoplex 1000/1600. Glucose and electrolytes for intravenous feeding.
Glucotard. Dietary aid for treatment of diabetes mellitus: see **Guar gum**.
Glurenorm. Oral antidiabetic: see **Gliquidone**.
Glutarol. Topical treatment for warts: see **Glutaraldehyde**.
Glutenex (b). **Gluten**-free dietary aid for coeliac disease.
Glutril. Oral hypoglycaemic: see **Glibornuride**.
Glyconon. Hypoglycaemic: see **Tolbutamide**.
Glykola. 'Tonic': see **Caffeine, Ferric salts, Glycerophosphate**.
Glymese. Hypoglycaemic: see **Chlorpropamide**.
Glypressin. Hormone: see **Terlipressin**.
Gonadotraphon. Hormone: see **Gonadotrophin**.
Gondafon. Oral hypoglycaemic: see **Glymidine**.
Graneodin. Antibiotic: see **Gramicidin, Neomycin**.

Gregoderm. Topical anti-infective/corticosteroid: see **Hydrocortisone Neomycin, Nystatin, Polymyxin B**.
Grisovin. Antifungal: see **Griseofulvin**.
GTN 300. Anti-anginal/vasodilator: see **Glyceryl trinitrate**.
Guanimycin susp. forte. Antibacterial/antidiarrhoeal: see **Dihydrostreptomycin, Kaolin, Sulphaguanidine**.
Guanor. Cough suppressant: see **Ammonium chloride, Diphenhydramine, Menthol**.
Guarem. Dietary aid for treatment of diabetes mellitus: see **Guar gum**.
Guarina. Dietary aid for diabetes mellitus: see **Guar Gum**.
Gynatren. Vaccine for recurrent trichomoniasis in females: see **Inactivated lactobacilli**.
Gyno-Daktarin. Local application for vaginal and penile fungal infections: see **Miconazole**.
Gynol II. Spermicidal jelly used for contraception: see **Nonoxynol**.
Gyno-Pevaryl. Antifungal for topical treatment of vaginal infections: see **Econazole**.
Gynovlar 21. Oral contraceptive: see **Ethinyloestradiol, Norethisterone**.

H

H.11. Polypeptide extract of male urine used in otherwise untreatable carcinoma.
Haelan. Topical corticosteroid: see **Flurandrenolone**.
Haelan-C. Topical corticosteroid/anti-infective: see **Clioquinol, Flurandrenolone**.
Haemaccel. Plasma expander: see **Gelatin, Sodium chloride**.
Halciderm. Topical corticosteroid for skin disorders: see **Halcinonide**.
Halcion. Hypnotic: see **Triazolam**.
Haldol. Tranquillizer: see **Haloperidol**.
Halin. Sustained-release nasal decongestant: see **Dexbrompheniramine, Pseudoephedrine**.
Halycitrol. Vitamins for injection: see **Vitamin A, Vitamin D**.
Hamarin. For gout: see **Allopurinol**.
Harmogen. Female sex hormones for deficiency states: see **Oestrone**.
Harmonyl (d). Antihypertensive: see **Deserpidine**.
Havapen (d). Antibiotic: see **Penamecillin**.
Haymine. For hay fever and similar allergic conditions: see **Chlorphenir-amine, Ephedrine**.
Hayphryn. Nasal decongestant spray: see **Phenylephrine, Thenyldiamine**.
H.B. Vax Vaccine for immunization against infective hepatitis (type B): see **Hepatitis B vaccine**.
Healonid. High-viscosity polymer solution for injection into eye during ophthalmic surgery: see **Sodium hyaluronate**.
Heminevrin. Sedative/hypnotic: see **Chlormethiazole**.

Hemoplex. Vitamin B mixture for deficiency state.
Hepacon B_{12}. For vitamin B_{12} deficiency and pernicious anaemia: see **Cyanocobalamin**.
Hepacon-B forte. For vitamin B_{12} and other deficiencies: see **Aneurine, Cyanocobalamin, Folic acid**.
Hepacon Liver injectable. For anaemia: see **Hydroxocobalamin, Liver extracts**.
Hepacon-Plex. For vitamin B deficiency: see **Aneurine, Cyanocobalamin, Nictonamide, Pantothenic acid, Pyridoxine, Riboflavine**.
Heparin retard. Anticoagulant formulated for intramuscular or deep subcutaneous injection: see **Heparin**.
Hepsal. Anticoagulant: see **Heparin**.
Herpid. Antiviral: see **Idoxuridine**.
Hespan. Plasma expander: see **Hetastarch**.
Hexopal. Peripheral vasodilator: see **Inositol nicotinate**.
Hibidil. Topical disinfectant to be used undiluted for hand and skin disinfection: see **Chlorhexidine**.
Hibiscrub. Antiseptic cleansing solution for pre-operative preparation of hands: see **Chlorhexidine**.
Hibisol. Topical disinfectant used undiluted for hand and skin disinfection: see **Chlorhexidine**.
Hibitane cream. Antiseptic for prevention of skin infection: see **Chlorhexidine**.
Hibitane lozenges. Antiseptic/local anaesthetic for infected sore throats: see **Benzocaine, Chlorhexidine**.
Hioxyl. Antiseptic for cleaning infected wounds: see **Hydrogen peroxide**.
Hiprex. Urinary anti-infective: see **Hexamine**.
Hirudoid. Anticoagulant cream for bruising associated with superficial thrombophlebitis or trauma: see **Heparin**.
Hismanal. Antihistamine: see **Astemizole**.
Histalix. Decongestant: see **Ammonium chloride, Diphenhydramine, Sodium citrate**.
Histryl. Antihistamine: see **Diphenylpyraline**.
Honvan. Synthetic sex hormone: see **Stilboestrol**.
Hormofemin cream. Synthetic sex hormone for pruritis, acne: see **Dienoestrol**.
Hormonin. Sex hormones for menopausal symptoms: see **Oestradiol, Oestriol, Oestrone**.
HRF. For diagnostic use in delayed sexual development and failure of pituitary gland function: see **Gonadorelin**.
Human Actraphane. Mixture of synthetic short- and long-acting human insulins: see **Insulin**.
Human Actrapid. Synthetic human crystalline insulin: see **Insulin**.
Human Initard 50/50. Semisynthetic human insulin made by biochemical conversion of porcine insulin: see **Insulin**.
Human Insulatard. Semisynthetic human insulin made by biochemical conversion of porcine insulin: see **Insulin**.

Human Mixtard 30/70. Semisynthetic human insulin made by biochemical conversion of porcine insulin: see **Insulin**.
Human Monotard. Long-acting synthetic human insulin (zinc suspension): see **Insulin**.
Human protaphane. Long-acting synthetic human (isophane) insulin: see **Insulin**.
Human Ultratard. Long-acting human insulin, prepared by modification of porcine insulin: see **Insulin**.
Human Velosulin. Semisynthetic human insulin made by biochemical conversion of porcine insulin: see **Insulin**.
Humotet. Purified human antitetanus immunoglobulin for passive immunization.
Humulin. Human insulins manufactured by genetic engineering using bacteria. Humulin S – soluble insulin, Humulin I – isophane insulin, Humulin M1/M2 – mixed soluble and isophane insulins, Humulin Zn – insulin zinc suspension: see **Insulin**.
Hyalase. Enzyme injection for addition to intramuscular/subcutaneous injection to aid absorption and decrease pain: see **Hyaluronidase**.
Hycal. High-calorie (carbohydrate), protein-free liquid for use in protein-free, low-electrolyte diet.
Hydergine. For impaired mental function in the elderly: see **Dihydroergotoxine**.
Hydrea. Cytotoxic: see **Hydroxyurea**.
Hydrenox. Diuretic: see **Hydroflumethiazide**.
Hydrocortistab. Corticosteroid for parenteral or topical use: see **Hydrocortisone**.
Hydrocortisyl. Corticosteroid cream for eczema and other skin conditions: see **Hydrocortisone**.
Hydrocortone. Corticosteroid for systemic or topical use: see **Hydrocortisone**.
Hydroderm. Corticosteroid/antibacterial cream for eczema: see **Bacitracin, Hydrocortisone, Neomycin**.
Hydromet. Antihypertensive/diuretic: see **Hydrochlorothiazide, Methyldopa**.
Hydrosaluric. Diuretic: see **Hydrochlorothiazide**.
Hygroton. Diuretic: see **Chlorthalidone**.
Hygroton K. As Hygroton plus **Potassium chloride** supplement.
Hypercal. Antihypertensive: see **Rauwolfia**.
Hypercal B (c). Antihypertensive/sedative: see **Amylobarbitone, Rauwolfia**.
Hypnomidate. Intravenous anaesthetic: see **Etomidate**.
Hypnovel. Intravenous sedative used before and during minor surgery: see **Midazolam**.
Hypon. Analgesic/antipyretic: see **Acetylsalicylic acid, Caffeine, Codeine**.
Hypotears. Eye drops for dry eyes: see **Polyethylene glycol, Polyvinyl alcohol**.
Hypovase. Antihypertensive: see **Prazosin**.
Hypurin isophane. Long-acting purified insulin: see **Insulin**.

Hypurin lente. Long-acting purified beef insulin (zinc suspension): see **Insulin**.

Hypurin neutral. Purified crystalline insulin: see **Insulin**.

Hypurin protamine zinc. Long-acting purified insulin: see **Insulin**.

I

Ibular. Anti-inflammatory/analgesic: see **Ibuprofen**.

Ibumetrin. Non-steroid anti-inflammatory/analgesic: see **Ibuprofen**.

Icthaband. Topical treatment for eczema: see **Zinc ichtammol**.

Idoxene. Eye ointment for treatment of herpetic keratitis (a viral infection of the cornea): see **Idoxuridine**.

Iliadin-mini. Nasal decongestant: see **Oxymetazoline**.

Ilonium. Protective, carminative ointment: see **Camphene, Colophony, Turpentine oil**.

Ilosone. Antibiotic: see **Erythromycin**.

Ilotycin. Antibiotic: see **Erythromycin**.

Ilube. Eye drops for dry eyes: see **Acetylcysteine, Hypromellose**.

Imbrilon. Non-steroid anti-inflammatory/analgesic: see **Indomethacin**.

Imferon. Haematinic: see **Iron dextran injection**.

Imodium. Antidiarrhoeal: see **Loperamide**.

Imunovir. For oral treatment of herpes simplex viral infections: see **Inosine pranabex**.

Imperacin. Antibiotic: see **Oxytetracycline**.

Imuran. Cytotoxic: see **Azathioprine**.

Inderal. Beta-adrenoceptor blocker: see **Propranolol**.

Inderal LA. Sustained-release antihypertensive: see **Propranolol**.

Inderetic. Antihypertensive: see **Bendrofluazide, Propranolol**.

Inderex. Antihypertensive: see **Bendrofluazide, Propranolol** (as in Inderal LA).

Indocid. Non-steroid anti-inflammatory/analgesic: see **Indomethacin**.

Indoflex. Non-steroid anti-inflammatory/analgesic: see **Indomethacin**.

Indolar. Non-steroid anti-inflammatory analgesic: see **Indomethacin**.

Indolar SR. Non-steroid anti-inflammatory/analgesic: see **Indomethacin**.

Indomod. Non-steroid anti-inflammatory/analgesic: see **Indomethacin**.

Innovace. Antihypertensive: see **Enalapril**.

Influvac. Inactivated influenza virus vaccine.

Initard. 50:50 long-acting purfied pork insulin mixture (50 percent neutral, 50 percent isophane): see **Insulin**.

Instillagel. Local anaesthetic/antiseptic gel for use in urethral catheterization and cystoscopy: see **Chlorhexidine, Lignocaine**.

Insulatard. Long-acting purified pork (isophane) insulin: see **Insulin**.

Intal. For asthma: see **Sodium cromoglycate**.

Intal compound. As Intal plus **Isoprenaline**.

Integrin. Anxiolytic: see **Oxypertine**.

Intraglobin. Concentrate of **Immunoglobulin** for patients with deficiency of this protein.
Intralgin. Rubefacient/local anaesthetic for muscle pain: see **Benzocaine, Salicylamide**.
Intralipid. High-energy source (fats) for intravenous feeding.
Intraval sodium. Short-acting intravenous barbiturate hypnotic for induction of anaesthesia: see **Thiopentone sodium**.
Intropin. Intravenous infusion for treatment of shock: see **Dopamine**.
Iodosorb. Iodine-releasing preparation used as antiseptic in skin ulcers.
Ionamin (c). Anti-obesity: see **Phentermine**.
Ionax Scrub. Soap substitute for use in acne: see **Benzalkonium**.
Ionil T. Shampoo for dermatitis of scalp: see **Benzalkonium, Coal tar**.
Ipral. Antimicrobial: see **Trimethoprim**.
Irofol C. Haematinic for prevention and treatment of anaemia of pregnancy: see **Ferrous sulphate, Folic acid, Vitamin C**.
Ironorm. Haematinic: see **Iron dextran injection**.
Ismelin. Antihypertensive: see **Guanethidine**.
Ismo 20. Antianginal: see **Isosorbide mononitrate**.
Iso-Autohaler. Aerosol bronchodilator: see **Isoprenaline**.
Iso-Brovon. Bronchodilator aerosol: see **Atropine methonitrate, Isoprenaline**.
Iso-Brovon Plus. Similar to Iso-Brovon, but higher dose of **Isoprenaline**.
Isogel. Purgative: see **Ispaghula**.
Isoket retard. Vasodilator: see **Isosorbide dinitrate**.
Isopto alkaline. Lubricant ('artificial tears') for dry eyes: see **Hypromellose**.
Isopto atropine. Long-acting mydriatic eye drops for cycloplegic refraction and uveitis: see **Atropine sulphate, Methylcellulose**.
Isopto carbachol. Miotic eye drops for glaucoma: see **Carbachol, Methylcellulose**.
Isopto carpine. Miotic eye drops for glaucoma: see **Methylcellulose, Pilocarpine**.
Isopto-Cetamide. Antibacterial eye drops: see **Sulphacetamide**.
Isopto epinal. Eye drops for glaucoma: see **Adrenaline**.
Isopto frin. Lubricant/decongestant for inflamed (but not infected) eye: see **Methylcellulose, Phenylephrine**.
Isopto plain. Lubricant ('artificial tears') for dry eyes: see **Hypromellose**.
Isordil. Antianginal: see **Isosorbide dinitrate**.
Isuprel. Sympathomimetic injection: see **Isoprenaline**.

J

Jectofer. For iron deficiency anaemia: see **Iron sorbitol injection**.
Jexin. Skeletal muscle relaxant: see **Tubocurarine**.

Juvel. Vitamin mixture: see **Aneurine, Calciferol, Nicotinamide, Pyridoxine, Riboflavine, Vitamin A, Vitamin C**.
Juvela. **Gluten**-free bread/cake mix.

K

Kabiglobulin. Injection of **Immunoglobulin**.
Kabikinase. Fibrinolytic: see **Streptokinase**.
Kalspare. Diuretic combination: see **Chlorthalidone, Triamterene**.
Kalten. Antihypertensive: see **Amiloride, Atenolol, Hydrochlorothiazide**.
Kamillosan oint. Topical preparation for sore skin: see **Resorcinol**.
Kannasyn. Antibiotic: see **Kanamycin**.
Kantrex. Antibiotic: see **Kanamycin**.
Kaodene. Antidiarrhoeal: see **Codeine, Kaolin**.
Kaopectate. Antidiarrhoeal: see **Kaolin**.
Kap-Amp (d). Antibiotic: see **Ampicillin**.
Kap-Ind (d). Non-steroid anti-inflammatory/analgesic: see **Indomethacin**.
Karvol. Inhalation for nasal congestion: see **Menthol**.
Kay-Cee-L. Potassium supplement: see **Potassium chloride**.
K-Contin. Potassium supplement: see **Potassium chloride**.
Kefadol. Antibiotic: see **Cephamandole**.
Keflex. Antibiotic: see **Cephalexin**.
Keflin. Antibotic: see **Cephalothin**.
Kefzol. Antibiotic: see **Cephazolin**.
Kelferon. For iron-deficiency anaemia: see **Ferrous glycine sulphate**.
Kelfizine W. Urinary anti-infective: see **Sulfametopyrazine**.
Kelfolate. For anaemia of pregnancy: see **Ferrous glycine sulphate, Folic acid**.
Kelocyanor. Antidote for cyanide poisoning: see **Cobalt tetracemate**.
Kemadrin. Antiparkinsonian: see **Procyclidine**.
Kemicetine (d). Antibiotic: see **Chloramphenicol**.
Kenalog. Corticosteroid injection for allergic conditions: see **Triamcinolone**.
Keralyt. Topical treatment for hyperkeratotic skin disorders: see **Salicylic acid**.
Kerecid. Local treatment for herpetic eye infections: see **Idoxuridine**.
Keri. Lotion for dry skin: see **Mineral oil**.
Kerlone. Antihypertensive: see **Betaxolol**.
Keromask (b). Concealing cream: see **Titanium dioxide**.
Kessar. For treatment of anovular infertility and breast cancer: see **Tamoxifen**.
Kest. Purgative: see **Magnesium sulphate, Phenolphthalein**.
Ketalar. Anaesthetic: see **Ketamine**.
Ketovite. Vitamin mixture: see **Acetomenaphthone, Aneurine, Folic acid, Nicotinamide, Pantothenic acid, Pyridoxine, Riboflavine, Vitamin C, Vitamin E**.

Kiditard. Sustained-release antidysrhythmic: see **Quinidine**.
Kinidin Durules. Sustained-release antidysrhythmic: see **Quinidine**.
KLN. Anti-diarrhoeal: see **Kaolin**.
Kloref. Effervescent potassium supplement: see **Potassium chloride**.
Klyx. Enema for purgation: see **Dioctyl sodium sulphosuccinate**.
Kolanticon. Antacid/antispasmodic: see **Aluminium hydroxide, Dicyclomine, Dimethicone, Magnesium oxide**.
Kolantyl. Antacid/antispasmodic: see **Aluminium hydroxide, Dicyclomine, Magnesium oxide**.
Konakion. For prothrombin deficiency: see **Phytomenadione**.

L

Labiton. 'Tonic': see **Aneurine, Caffeine, *para*-Aminobenzoic acid**.
Labophylline (d). Bronchodilator: see **Theophylline**.
Laboprin. Anti-inflammatory/analgesic: see **Acetylsalicylic acid**.
Labosept. Oral antiseptic: see **Dequalinium**.
Labrocol. Antihypertensive: see **Labetalol**.
Lacri-Lube. Lubricant eye ointment for dry eyes: see **Hydrous wool fat, Liquid paraffin**.
Lacticare. Skin lotion: see **Lactic acid, Sodium pyrrolidone-carboxylate**.
Ladropen. Antibiotic: see **Flucloxacillin**.
Laevulfex. Intravenous energy source: see **Laevulose**.
Lamprene. Antileprosy: see **Clofazimine**.
Lance B & C (d). Vitamin supplement: see **Aneurine, Nicotinamide, Pyridoxine, Riboflavine, Vitamin C**.
Lanitop. For cardiac failure: see **Medigoxin**.
Lanoxin. For cardiac failure: see **Digoxin**.
Lanvis. Cytotoxic: see **Thioguanine**.
Laracor. Beta-adrenoceptor blocker: see **Oxprenolol**.
Laractone. Diuretic: see **Spironolactone**.
Laraflex. Non-steroid anti-inflammatory/analgesic: see **Naproxen**.
Laratrim. Antibiotic: see **Co-trimoxazole**.
Largactil. Major tranquillizer/anti-emetic/antivertigo: see **Chlorpromazine**.
Larodopa. Antiparkinsonian: see **Levodopa**.
Lasikal. Diuretic with potassium supplement: see **Frusemide, Potassium chloride**.
Lasilactone. Combination of two diuretics with different modes of action for use in refractory oedema: see **Frusemide, Spironolactone**.
Lasipressin. Antihypertensive: see **Frusemide, Penbutolol**.
Lasix. Diuretic: see **Frusemide**.
Lasix + K. Diuretic/potassium supplement: see **Frusemide, Potassium chloride**.
Lasma. Sustained-release bronchodilator: see **Theophylline**.

Lasonil. Topical treatment for soft tissue injury: see **Heparin, Hyaluronidase**.
Laxoberal. Purgative: see **Sodium picosulphate**.
Ledclair. For heavy metal poisoning: see **Sodium calcium edetate**.
Ledercort. Corticosteroid for topical or systemic use: see **Triamcinolone**.
Lederfen. Non-steroid anti-inflammatory/analgesic: see **Fenbufen**.
Lederkyn. Antibacterial: see **Sulphamethoxypyridazine**.
Ledermycin. Antibiotic: see **Demethylchlortetracycline**.
Lederplex. Vitamin B mixture: see **Aneurine, Cyanocobalmin, Niacinamide, Pantothenic acid, Pyridoxine, Riboflavine**.
Lederspan. Corticosteroid injection: see **Triamcinolone**.
Lejfibre. High-fibre biscuits for constipation: see **Bran**.
Lejguar. Flour for stabilization of blood glucose levels in diabetes mellitus: see **Guar flour**.
Lenium (b). Shampoo for dandruff: see **Selenium sulphide**.
Lentard. Mixture of long-acting purified beef and pork (zinc suspension) insulins: see **Insulin**.
Lentizol. Sustained release. Antidepressant: see **Amitriptyline**.
Leo K. Slow-release potassium supplement: see **Potassium chloride**.
Lergoban. Anti-allergic: see **Diphenylpyraline**.
Leukeran. Cytotoxic: see **Chlorambucil**.
Levius. Anti-inflammatory/analgesic: see **Acetylsalicylic acid**.
Levophed. Vasoconstrictor: see **Noradrenaline**.
Lexotan. Anxiolytic: see **Bromazepam**.
Lexpec. Haematinic: see **Folic acid**.
Libanil. Oral hypoglycaemic: see **Glibenclamide**.
Libraxin. Anxiolytic antispasmodic: see **Chlordiazepoxide, Clidinium**.
Librium. Anxiolytic: see **Chlordiazepoxide**.
Limbritol 10 and 5. Antidepressant/anxiolytic: see **Amitriptyline, Chlordiazepoxide**.
Limclair. Increases calcium excretion: see **Sodium edetate**.
Lincocin. Antibiotic: see **Lincomycin**.
Linctifed. Decongestant/mucolytic: see **Codeine, Guaiphenesin, Pseudoephedrine, Triprolidine**.
Lingraine. Vasoconstrictor for migraine: see **Ergotamine**.
Lioresal. Muscle relaxant: see **Baclofen**.
Lipoflavonoid. Multiple vitamins preparation for Ménière's disease.
Lipotriad. Multiple vitamins for retinal degeneration.
Liquifilm tears. Lubricant eye drops for dry eyes: see **Polyvinyl alcohol**.
Liquigen (b). Milk substitute for malabsorption states containing medium-chain triglycerides.
Liskonum. Antidepressant: see **Lithium salts**.
Litarex. Sustained-release antidepressant: see **Lithium salts**.
Loasid. Antacid: see **Aluminium hydroxide, Dimethicone, Magnesium hydroxide**.
Lobak. Analgesic: see **Chlormezanone, Paracetamol**.
Locabiotal. Topical antibiotic for infections of upper respiratory tract: see **Fusafungine**.

Locan. Topical anaesthetic cream: see **Amethocaine, Amylocaine, Cinchocaine**.
Locasol (b). Low-calcium food substitute for calcium intolerance.
Locoid. Topical corticosteroid for eczema and other skin conditions: see **Hydrocortisone**.
Locoid C. Topical corticosteroid/anti-infective: see **Chlorquinadol, Hydrocortisone**.
Locorten/Vioform. Topical corticosteroid/anti-infective for skin or ears: see **Clioquinol, Flumethasone**.
Lodine. Non-steroid anti-inflammatory/analgesic: see **Etodolac**.
Loestrin 20. Oral contraceptive: see **Ethinyloestradiol, Norethisterone**.
Lofenalac (b). Dietary substitute for phenylketonuria.
Logynon. Oral contraceptive: see **Ethinyloestradiol, Levonorgestrel**.
Lomodex 40 and 70. Plasma expanders: see **Dextrans**.
Lomotil. Antidiarrhoeal: see **Atropine, Diphenoxylate**.
Loniten. Antihypertensive: see **Minoxidil**.
Lopresor. Beta-adrenoceptor blocker: see **Metoprolol**.
Lopresor S.R. Sustained-release formulation of Lopresor.
Lopresoretic. Antihypertensive: see **Chlorthalidone, Metoprolol**.
Loramet. Hypnotic: see **Lormetazepam**.
Lorexane. Lotion for head lice: see **Gamma-benzene hexachloride**.
Lotussin. Cough linctus/decongestant: see **Dextromethorphan, Diphenhydramine, Ephedrine, Guaiphenesin**.
Ludiomil. Antidepressant: see **Maprotiline**.
Lugacin. Antibiotic: see **Gentamicin**.
Luminal (c). Anticonvulsant/hypnotic: see **Phenobarbitone**.
Lurselle. Lowers blood cholesterol concentrations in hypercholesterolaemia: see **Probucol**.

M

Maalox. Antacid: see **Aluminium hydroxide, Magnesium hydroxide**.
Macrodantin. Antibacterial: see **Nitrofurantoin**.
Macrodex. Plasma expander: see **Dextrans**.
Madopar. Antiparkinsonian: see **Benserazide, Levodopa**.
Madribon. Antibacterial: see **Sulphadimethoxine**.
Magnapen. Antibiotic: see **Ampicillin, Flucloxacillin**.
Malarivon. Antimalarial elixir: see **Chloroquine**.
Malatex. Keratolytic cream/solution for removal of thickened, dry skin: see **Benzoic acid, Malic acid, Propylene glycol, Salicylic acid**.
Malinal. Antacid: see **Almasilate**.
Malix. Hypoglycaemic: see **Glibenclamide**.
Maloprim. Antimalarials for prophylaxis: see **Dapsone, Pyrimethamine**.
Mandelamine (d). Urinary anti-infective: see **Hexamine mandelate**.
Mansil. Anti-infective: see **Oxamniquine**.

Manusept. Topical antiseptic: see **Triclosan**.
Marboran. Antiviral: see **Methisazone**.
Marcain. Local anaesthetic injection: see **Bupivacaine**.
Marevan. Oral anticoagulant: see **Warfarin**.
Marplan. Antidepressant (monoamine oxidase inhibitor): see **Isocarboxazid**.
Marsilid. Antidepressant (monoamine oxidase inhibitor: see **Iproniazid**.
Marvelon. Oral contraceptive: see **Desogestrel, Ethinyloestradiol**.
Masse. Soothing cream for nipples during lactation: see **Allantoin, Aminoacridine**.
Masteril. Sex hormone for treatment of neoplasms of the breast: see **Drostanolone**.
Maxamaid (b). Phenylalanine-free mixture of **Amino acids** for phenylketonuric patients.
Maxidex. Corticosteroid eye drops for non-infective, inflammatory conditions: see **Dexamethasone**.
Maxipro HBV (b). Source of protein for malabsorption states.
Maxitrol. Corticosteroid/antibiotic eye drops/ointment. see **Dexamethasone, Neomycin, Polymyxin B**.
Maxolon. Anti-emetic: see **Metoclopramide**.
Maxtrex. Cytotoxic: see **Methotrexate**.
MCT (1) and MCT Oil (b). Dietary substitutes containing triglycerides. For use in impaired fat absorption.
Medicoal. Oral adsorbant for treatment of acute poisoning and drug overdose: see **Activated charcoal**.
Medihaler-Duo. Bronchodilator aerosol: see **Isoprenaline, Phenylephrine**.
Medihaler-Epi. Bronchodilator aerosol: see **Adrenaline**.
Medihaler-Ergotamine (d). Aerosol inhalation for migraine: see **Ergotamine**.
Medihaler-Iso/Medihaler Iso-Forte. Bronchodilator aerosol: see **Isoprenaline**.
Medilave. Oral disinfectant: see **Benzocaine, Cetylpyridinium**.
Medised. Analgesic/sedative: see **Paracetamol, Promethazine**.
Meditar. For psoriasis: see **Coal tar**.
Medocodene. Analgesic: see **Co-codamol**.
Medomet. Antihypertensive: see **Methyldopa**.
Medrone. Corticosteroid: see **Methylprednisolone**.
Medrone acne lotion. Topical treatment for acne: see **Aluminium chlorohydrate, Methylprednisolone, Sulphur**.
Mefoxin. Antibiotic: see **Cefoxitin**.
Megace. Sex hormone: see **Megestrol**.
Megaclor. Antibiotic: see **Clomocycline**.
Melitase (d). Oral hypoglycaemic: see **Chlorpropamide**.
Melleril. Tranquillizer: see **Thioridazine**.
Menophase. Sex hormones for menopausal disorders: see **Mestranol, Norethisterone**.
Meprate. Anxiolytic: see **Meprobamate**.
Meptid. Analgesic: see **Meptazinol**.

Merbentyl. Anticholinergic for gastro-intestinal colic: see **Dicyclomine**.
Merieux Tetavax. Purified tetanus toxoid for active immunization against tetanus.
Merital (d). Antidepressant: see **Nomifensine**.
Merocaine. Antiseptic/local anaesthetic lozenge for painful mouth conditions: see **Benzocaine, Cetylpyridinium**.
Merocet. Antiseptic mouthwash or lozenges: see **Cetylpyridinium**.
Meruvax 11. Live attenuated vaccine for immunization against German measles: see **Rubella vaccine**.
Mestinon. Anticholinesterase: see **Pyridostigmine**.
Metabolic Mineral Mixture (b). Dietary mineral supplement.
Metamucil. Purgative: see **Ispaghula**.
Metanium. Soothing, protective ointment and powder for nappy rash and other macerated skin conditions: see **Titanium dioxide**.
Metatone. 'Tonic': see **Aneurine, Glycerophosphates**.
Metenix 5. Diuretic: see **Metolazone**.
Meterfer. Haematinic: see **Ferrous fumarate**.
Meterfolic. Haematinic: see **Ferrous fumarate, Folic acid**.
Metopirone. Used in test of pituitary function: see **Metyrapone**.
Metosyn. Topical corticosteroid for skin disorders: see **Fluocinonide**.
Metox. Anti-emetic: see **Metoclopromide**.
Metrodin. Hormone: see **Urofollitrophin**.
Metrolyl. Antimicrobial: see **Metronidazole**.
Mevilin-L. Live attenuated **Measles vaccine**.
Mexitil. Antidysrhythmic: see **Mexiletine**.
Mexitil Perlongets. Sustained-release form of Mexitil: see **Mexiletine**.
M F V-Ject. Influenza vaccine for immunization.
Micolette. Laxative enema: see **Glycerol, Sodium citrate, Sodium lauryl sulphoacetate**.
Micralax. Purgative enema: see **Sodium alkyl sulphoacetate, Sodium citrate, Sorbic acid**.
Microgynon 30. Oral contraceptive: see **Ethinyloestradiol, Norgestrel**.
Micro K. Slow-release potassium supplement: see **Potassium chloride**.
Micronor. Oral contraceptive: see **Norethisterone**.
Microval. Oral contraceptive: see **Levonorgestrel**.
Mictral. For urinary tract infections: see **Nalidixic acid**.
Midamor. Diuretic: see **Amiloride**.
Midrid. For headache, migraine: see **Dichloralphenazone, Isometheptene, Paracetamol**.
Migen. Extract of house dust mite for allergy densitization.
Migraleve. For migraine: see **Buclizine, Codeine, Dioctyl sodium sulphosuccinate, Paracetamol**.
Migravess. Soluble analgesic/anti-emetic for migraine. **Metoclopramide** aids drug absorption by relief of the gastric stasis which can occur during a migraine attack as well as acting as an anti-emetic: see **Acetylsalicylic acid, Metoclopramide**.
Migril. Vasoconstrictor for migraine: see **Caffeine, Cyclizine, Ergotamine**.
Millophyline (d). Cardiac stimulant/bronchodilator: see **Etamiphyllin**.

Minafen (b). Dietary preparation for phenylketonuria.
Minamino. Mixture of minerals and vitamins for deficiency states.
Minihep. Subcutaneous injection for thromboembolic disease: see **Heparin**.
Mini-i-jet. Sympathomimetic: see **Adrenaline**.
Minilyn. Oral contraceptive: see **Ethinyloestradiol, Lynoestrenol**.
Minims. Single dose ophthalmic preparations.
Minocin. Antibiotic: see **Minocycline**.
Minodiab. Oral hypoglycaemic: see **Glipizide**.
Minovlar. Oral contraceptive: see **Ethinyloestradiol, Norethisterone**.
Mintezol. Anthelmintic: see **Thiabendazole**.
Miochol. Solution for intra-ocular irrigation during eye surgery: see **Acetylcholine**.
Miol. Soothing lotion/cream for irritated skin conditions.
Miraxid. Antibiotic: see **Pivampicillin, Pivmecillinam**.
Mithracin. Cytotoxic: see **Mithramycin**.
Mitomycin C Kyowa. Cytotoxic: see **Mitomycin**.
Mitoxana. Cytotoxic: see **Ifosfamide**.
Mixogen. Sex hormones for menopausal symptoms, suppression of lactation: see **Ethinyloestradiol, Methyltestosterone**.
Mixtard. 30:70 long-acting purified pork insulin mixture (30 percent neutral, 70 percent isophane): see **Insulin**.
Mobilan. Non-steroid anti-inflammatory/analgesic: see **Indomethacin**.
Modecate. Long-acting tranquillizer injection: see **Fluphenazine**.
Moditen. Tranquillizer: see **Fluphenazine**.
Moditen enanthate. Long-acting tranquillizer injection: see **Fluphenazine**.
Modrenal. Used to suppress secretion of adrenal cortical hormones: see **Trilostane**.
Moducren. Antihypertensive: see **Amiloride, Hydrochlorothiazide, Timolol**.
Moduret 25. Diuretic combination: see **Amiloride, Hydrochlorothiazide**.
Moduretic. Diuretic combination. Available as solution for patients who cannot swallow tablets: see **Amiloride, Hydrochlorothiazide**.
Mogadon. Hypnotic: see **Nitrazepam**.
Molcer. Drops to soften ear wax: see **Dioctyl sodium sulphosuccinate**.
Molipaxin. Antidepressant: see **Trazodone**.
Monaspor. Antimicrobial injection: see **Cefsoludin**.
Monistat. Topical antifungal: see **Miconazole**.
Monit. Antianginal: see **Isosorbide mononitrate**.
Mono-Cedocard. Antianginal: see **Isosorbide mononitrate**.
Monodral. Anticholinergic for reducing gastric motility and secretion: see **Penthienate**.
Monoparin. Anticoagulant: see **Heparin**.
Monophane. Long-acting purified beef (isophane) insulin: see **Insulin**.
Monophytol. Topical antifungal: see **Boric acid, Chlorbutol, Salicylic acid, Undecenoic acid**.
Monotard. Long-acting purified pork insulin (zinc suspension): see **Insulin**.

Monotrim. Antimicrobial: see **Trimethoprim**.
Morhulin. Topical preparation for abrasions, skin ulcers: see **Cetrimide, Dakin's solution, Zinc oxide**.
Morsep. Topical preparation for nappy rash: see **Cetrimide, Dakin's solution**.
Motilium. Anti-emetic: see **Domperidone**.
Motipress. Sedative/antidepressant: see **Fluphenazine, Nortriptyline**.
Motival. Sedative/antidepressant: see **Fluphenazine, Nortriptyline**.
Motrin. Non-steroid anti-inflammatory/analgesic: see **Ibuprofen**.
Movelat. Rubefacient: see **Corticosteroid, Salicylic acid**.
Moxalactam. Antibiotic: see **Latamoxef**.
MST continus (c). Sustained-release oral narcotic analgesic: see **Morphine**.
M.S.U.D. Aid (b). Dietary aid for maple syrup urine disease.
Mucaine. Antacid for oesophageal pain: see **Aluminium hydroxide, Magnesium hydroxide, Oxethazaine**.
Mucodyne. Mucolytic: see **Carbocysteine**.
Mucogel. Antacid: see **Aluminium hydroxide, Magnesium hydroxide**.
Mucolex. Mucolytic: see **Carbocysteine**.
Multibionta. Intravenous vitamins: see **Aneurine, Nicotinamide, Pantothenic acid, Pyridoxine, Riboflavine, Vitamin A, Vitamin C, Vitamin E**.
Multilind. Antifungal cream: see **Nystatin**.
Multiparin. Anticoagulant: see **Heparin**.
Multivite. Vitamin mixture: see **Aneurine, Calciferol, Vitamin A, Vitamin C**.
Mumpsvax. Live mumps virus vaccine.
Muripsin. Preparation of hydrochloric acid and **Pepsin** for deficient gastric secretion.
Myambutol. Anti-tuberculosis: see **Ethambutol**.
Mycardol. Antianginal: see **Pentaerythritol tetranitrate**.
Mycifradin. Antibiotic: see **Neomycin**.
Myciguent. Topical antibiotic: see **Neomycin**.
Mycil. Topical antifungal: see **Chlorphenesin**.
Mycolactine. Purgative: see **Aloes**.
Mycota. Topical antifungal: see **Undecenoic acid**.
Mydriacyl. Mydriatic/cycloplegic eye drops: see **Tropicamide**.
Mydrilate. Mydriatic/cycloplegic eye drops: see **Cyclopentolate**.
Myelobromol. Cytotoxic: see **Mitobronitol**.
Mygdalon. Anti-emetic: see **Metoclopramide**.
Myleran. Cytotoxic: see **Busulphan**.
Mynah. Anti-tuberculosis: see **Ethambutol, Isoniazid**.
Myocrisin. Gold injection for rheumatoid arthritis: see **Aurothiomalate sodium**.
Myolgin. Analgesic: see **Acetylsalicylic acid, Caffeine, Codeine, Paracetamol**.
Myotonine chloride. Produces gut and bladder emptying: see **Bethanechol**.
Mysoline. Anticonvulsant: see **Primidone**.

Mysteclin. Antibiotic/antifungal: see **Nystatin, Tetracycline**.
Mytelase. For myasthenia gravis: see **Ambenonium**.

N

Nacton/Nacton forte. Anticholinergic for peptic ulcers: see **Poldine**.
Nalcrom. For ulcerative colitis: see **Sodium cromoglycate**.
Naprosyn. Non-steroid anti-inflammatory/analgesic: see **Naproxen**.
Napsalgesic. Analgesic: see **Acetylsalicylic acid, Dextropropoxyphene**.
Narcan. Narcotic antagonist: see **Naloxone**.
Nardil. Antidepressant (monoamine oxidase inhibitor): see **Phenelzine**.
Narphen (c). Analgesic: see **Phenazocine**.
Naseptin. Antiseptic/antibacterial cream for topical use in nasal carriers of staphylococci: see **Chlorhexidine, Neomycin**.
Natirose. Antianginal: see **Ethylmorphine, Glyceryl trinitrate, Hyoscyamine**.
Natrilix. Antihypertensive: see **Indapamide**.
Natuderm. Bland protective ('barrier') cream.
Natulan. Cytotoxic: see **Procarbazine**.
Navidrex. Diuretic: see **Cyclopenthiazide**.
Navidrex-K. As Navidrex plus **Potassium chloride** in slow-release wax core.
Naxogin/Naxogin 500. Antiprotozoal: see **Nimorazole**.
Nebcin. Antibiotic: see **Tobramycin**.
Negram. Antibacterial: see **Nalidixic acid**.
Nembutal (c). Hypnotic: see **Pentobarbitone**.
Neobacrin oint. Topical anti-infective: see **Bacitracin, Neomycin**.
Neocon 1/35. Oral contraceptive: see **Ethinyloestradiol, Norethisterone**.
Neo-cortef. Topical corticosteroid/antibacterial ointment/lotion/drops: see **Hydrocortisone, Neomycin**.
Neo-Cytamen. Vitamin: see **Hydroxocobalamin**.
Neogest. Oral contraceptive: see **Norgestrel**.
Neo-Mercazole. Antithyroid: see **Carbimazole**.
Neo-Naclex. Diuretic: see **Bendrofluazide**.
Neo-Naclex-K. As Neo-Naclex plus **Potassium chloride** in slow-release matrix.
Neophryn. Nasal decongestant: see **Phenylephrine**.
Neoplatin. Cytotoxic: see **Cisplatin**.
Neosporin. Antibacterial eye drops: see **Gramicidin, Neomycin, Polymyxin B**.
Nepenthe (c). Narcotic analgesic: see **Morphine**.
Nephril. Diuretic: see **Polythiazide**.
Nericur. Gel for topical treatment of acne: see **Benzoyl peroxide**.
Nerisone. Corticosteroid cream for skin conditions: see **Diflucortolone**.
Nestosyl. Topical ointment for painful, itchy skin conditions: see **Benzocaine, Butyl aminobenzoate, Hexachlorphane, Resorcinol, Zinc oxide**.

Nethaprin Dospan. Slow-release bronchodilator: see **Bufylline, Etafedrine, Doxylamine, Phenylephrine**.

Nethaprin expectorant. As Nethaprin minus phenylephrine but plus **Guaiphenesin** as expectorant.

Netillin. Antibiotic: see **Netilmicin**.

Neulactil. Antipsychotic: see **Pericyazine**.

Neulente. Purified long-acting insulin zinc suspension: see **Insulin**.

Neuphane. Purified long-acting (isophane) insulin: see **Insulin**.

Neurodyne. Analgesic: see **Co-codamol**.

Neusulin. Purified crystalline insulin: see **Insulin**.

Neutradonna. Antacid/anticholinergic for peptic ulcers: see **Aluminium antacids, Belladonna extract**.

Neutraphylline. Bronchodilator: see **Diprophylline**.

Nezcaam. Nasal decongestant: see **Guaiphenesin, Phenylpropanolamine**.

Nidazol. Antimicrobial: see **Metronidazole**.

Niferex. Haematinic: see **Polysaccharide–iron complex**.

Nilstim. Anti-obesity bulk agent: see **Methylcellulose**.

Nipride. Intravenous antihypertensive: see **Sodium nitroprusside**.

Nitoman. For treatment of chorea and related disorders: see **Tetrabenazine**.

Nitrados. Hypnotic: see **Nitrazepam**.

Nitrocine. Antianginal/vasodilator injection. Used as infusion to prevent myocardial ischaemia (e.g., in cardiac surgery or unstable angina): see **Glyceryl trinitrate**.

Nitrocontin. Antianginal: see **Glyceryl trinitrate**.

Nitrolingual. Vasodilator oral spray for symptomatic relief of angina: see **Glyceryl trinitrate**.

Nivaquine. Antimalarial: see **Chloroquine**.

Nivemycin. Antibiotic for oral and topical use: see **Neomycin**.

Nizoral. Antifungal: see **Ketoconazole**.

Nobrium. Anxiolytic: see **Medazepam**.

Noctamid. Hypnotic: see **Lormetazepam**.

Noctec. Hypnotic: see **Chloral hydrate**.

Noctesed. Hypnotic: see **Nitrazepam**.

Noltam. For treatment of anovular infertility and breast cancer: see **Tamoxifen**.

Noludar (c). Hypnotic: see **Methyprylone**.

Nolvadex. For treatment of anovular infertility and breast cancer: see **Tamoxifen**.

Nolvadex-D. As Nolvadex formulated for once-daily dosage: see **Tamoxifen**.

Noradran. Bronchodilator expectorant: see **Guaiphenesin, Diphenhydramine, Diprophylline, Ephedrine**.

Noratex. Cream for bed sores: see **Cod liver oil, Kaolin** (light), **Talc, Zinc oxide**.

Norcuron. Muscle relaxant: see **Vecuronium**.

Nordox. Antibiotic: see **Doxycycline**.

Norflex. Slow-release muscle relaxant: see **Orphenadrine**.

Norgesic. Muscle relaxant/analgesic: see **Paracetamol, Orphenadrine**.
Norgeston. Oral contraceptive: see **Levonorgestrel**.
Norgotin. Decongestant/anaesthetic/anti-infective for inflammation of outer ear: see **Amethocaine, Chlorhexidine, Ephedrine**.
Noriday. Oral contraceptive: see **Norethisterone**.
Norimin. Oral contraceptive: see **Ethinyloestradiol, Norethisterone**.
Norinyl-1/Norinyl-1/28. Oral contraceptives: see **Mestranol, Norethisterone**.
Norisen. Pollen extracts for desensitization in asthma and hay fever.
Noristerat. Depot contraceptive: see **Norethisterone**.
Norlestrin (d). For menstrual disorders: see **Ethinyloestradiol, Norethisterone**.
Normacol. Purgative: see **Frangula, Sterculia**.
Normasol Undine. Single-dose ophthalmic preparation of **Sodium chloride**.
Normax. Purgative: see **Co-danthrusate**.
Normetic. Diuretic combination: see **Amiloride, Hydrochlorothiazide**.
Normison. Hypnotic: see **Temazepam**.
Norval. Antidepressant: see **Mianserin**.
Novantrone. Cytotoxic: see **Mitozantrone**.
Noxyflex S. Anti-infective for instillation in bladder or other body cavities: see **Noxythioline**.
Noxyflex with amethocaine. As Noxyflex S plus **Amethocaine** as local anaesthetic.
Nozinan. Antipsychotic: see **Methotrimeprazine**.
Nubain. Analgesic: see **Nalbuphine**.
Nuelin. Bronchodilator: see **Theophylline**.
Nu K. Potassium supplement: see **Potassium chloride**.
Nulacin. Antacid: see **Calcium and Magnesium antacids**.
Numotac. Bronchodilator: see **Isoetharine**.
Nupercaine (d). Topical skin anaesthetic: see **Cinchocaine**.
Nu-Seals Aspirin. Enteric-coated analgesic: see **Acetylsalicylic acid**.
Nutracel 400/800. Glucose and electrolytes for intravenous feeding.
Nutramigen (b). Dietary aid for lactose intolerance, galactosaemia.
Nutraplus. Topical cream for dry skin: see **Urea**.
Nutrizym. For use in pancreatic deficiency: see **Pancreatic enzymes**.
Nybadex. Topical antifungal/anti-inflammatory: see **Hydrocortisone, Nystatin**.
Nydrane. Anticonvulsant: see **Beclamide**.
Nyspes. Antifungal pessaries: see **Nystatin**.
Nystadermal (d). Topical antifungal/anti-inflammatory: see **Nystatin, Triamcinolone**.
Nystaform. Cream or ointment for topical treatment of fungal skin infections due to *Candida* spp.: see **Chlorhexidine, Nystatin**.
Nystaform-HC. Topical anti-infective/anti-inflammatory: see **Chlorhexidine, Hydrocortisone, Nystatin**.
Nystan. Antifungal: see **Nystatin**.
Nystavescent. Vaginal antifungal: see **Nystatin**.

O

Octapressin. Vasoconstrictor: see **Felypressin**.

Octovit. Multi-vitamin and mineral supplement: see **Ascorbic acid, Cyanocobalamin, Nicotinamide, Pyridoxine, Riboflavine, Thiamine, Tocopherol, Vitamin A;** plus **Calcium, Iron, Magnesium, Zinc**.

Ocusert Pilo. Topical sustained-release treatment for glaucoma. The drug is contained within a membrane in single dose units which are placed under the eyelid: see **Pilocarpine**.

Ocusol. Antibacterial eye drops: see **Sulphacetamide**.

Omnopon (c). Narcotic analgesic: see **Papaveretum**.

Omnopon-Scopolamine (c). Norcotic analgesic/anticholinergic for use prior to operation: see **Papaveretum, Hyoscine hydrobromide**.

Oncovin. Cytotoxic: see **Vincristine**.

One-Alpha. Hormone: see **Alpha-calcidol**.

Operidine (c). Narcotic analgesic: see **Phenoperidine**.

Ophthaine. Topical ophthalmic anaesthetic: see **Proxymetacaine**.

Ophthalmadine. Local treatment for herpetic eye infections: see **Idox-uridine**.

Opilon. Peripheral vasodilator: see **Thymoxamine**.

Opobyl. Purgative: see **Aloes, Bile salts, Podophyllin**.

Opren (d). Non-steroid anti-inflammatory/analgesic: see **Benoxaprofen**.

Opticrom. Eye drops for allergic conjunctivitis: see **Sodium cromoglycate**.

Optimax. Antidepressant: see **Tryptophan**.

Optimine. Antihistamine: see **Azatadine**.

Opulets. Single-dose ophthalmic preparations.

Orabase. Topical inert protective application for skin and mucosae.

Orabolin. Anabolic steroid: see **Ethyloestrenol**.

Oradexon. Corticosteroid: see **Dexamethasone**.

Orahesive. Topical inert protective powder for skin and mucosae.

Oral B. Oral disinfectant: see **Cetylpyridinium, Lignocaine**.

Oralcer. For oral ulcers: see **Clioquinol**.

Oraldene. Rinse for oral infections: see **Hexetidine**.

Orap. Tranquillizer: see **Pimozide**.

Orbenin. Antibiotic: see **Cloxacillin**.

Organidin. Expectorant containing iodine.

Orimeten. Cytotoxic: see **Aminoglutethimide**.

Orlest 21 (d). Oral contraceptive: see **Ethinyloestradiol, Norethisterone**.

Orovite. Vitamin mixture: see **Aneurine, Nicotinamide, Pyridoxine, Vitamin C**.

Ortho-Creme. Spermicidal cream: see **Nonoxynol, Ricinoleic acid, Sodium lauryl sulphate**.

Ortho-Forms. Spermicidal pessary.

Ortho-Gynol. Spermicidal jelly.

Ortho-Novin. Oral contraceptive: see **Mestranol, Norethisterone**.

Orthoxicol. Cough suppressant: see **Codeine, Methoxyphenamine**.

Orthoxine. Bronchodilator: see **Methoxyphenamine**.

Orudis. Non-steroid anti-inflammatory/analgesic: see **Ketoprofen**.
Oruvail. Sustained-release non-steroid anti-inflammatory/analgesic: see **Ketoprofen**.
Osmitrol. Diuretic for intravenous infusion: see **Mannitol**.
Osmolite (b). Liquid feed for enteral absorption.
Ospolot (d). Anticonvulsant: see **Sulthiame**.
Ossopan. Source of calcium and fluoride for bone and dental states.
Otosporin. Antibiotic/anti-inflammatory ear drops: see **Hydrocortisone, Neomycin, Polymyxin B**.
Ototrips. Antibiotic topical preparation for ear: see **Bacitracin, Polymyxin B**.
Otrivine. Nasal decongestant: see **Xylometazoline**.
Otrivine-Antistin. Topical antihistamine/vasoconstrictor anti-allergic preparation: see **Antazoline, Xylometazoline**.
Ouabaine Arnaud. For treatment of cardiac failure and abnormal heart rhythms: see **Ouabain**.
Ovestin. Female sex hormone for deficiency states: see **Oestriol**.
Ovol (d). Antispasmodic: see **Dicyclomine**.
Ovran. Oral contraceptive: see **Ethinyloestradiol, Norgestrel**.
Ovranette. Oral contraceptive: see **Ethinyloestradiol, Norgestrel**.
Ovulen (d). Oral contraceptive: see **Ethynodiol, Mestranol**.
Ovysmen. Oral contraceptive: see **Ethinyloestradiol, Norethisterone**.
Oxanid. Anxiolytic: see **Oxazepam**.
Oxymycin. Antibiotic: see **Oxytetracycline**.

P

Pabrinex. Vitamin injection: see **Vitamin B, Vitamin C**.
Pacitron. Antidepressant: see **Tryptophan**.
Paedo-Sed. Hypnotic/analgesic: see **Dichloralphenazone, Paracetamol**.
Palaprin forte. Non-steroid anti-inflammatory/analgesic: see **Aloxiprin**.
Paldesic. Analgesic elixir: see **Paracetamol**.
Palfium (c). Narcotic analgesic: see **Dextromoramide**.
Paludrine. Antimalarial: see **Proguanil**.
Pamergan (c). Premedication combination containing narcotic analgesic: see **Pethidine, Promethazine**.
Pameton (d). Analgesic with antidote against overdose: see **Methionine, Paracetamol**.
Panadeine. Analgesic: see **Co-codamol**.
Panadeine Forte. Analgesic: see **Paracetamol**.
Panadol. Analgesic: see **Codeine, Paracetamol**.
Panar. For cystic fibrosis: see **Pancreatic enzymes**.
Panasorb. Analgesic: see **Paracetamol**.
Pancrease. See **Pancreatic enzymes**.
Pancreolauryl Test. Dye for testing pancreatic function: see **Flurescein**.

Pancrex/Pancrex V/Pancrex V Forte. For use in pancreatic deficiency: see **Pancreatin**.

Panoxyl 5 and 10. Topical treatment for acne: see **Benzoyl peroxide**.

Paracodol. Effervescent analgesic/antipyretic: see **Codeine, Paracetamol**.

Paradeine. Analgesic: see **Codeine, Paracetamol, Phenolphthalein**.

Parahypon. Analgesic/antipyretic: see **Caffeine, Codeine, Paracetamol**.

Parake. Analgesic/antipyretic: see **Co-codamol**.

Paralgin (d). Analgesic/antipyretic: see **Caffeine, Codeine, Paracetamol**.

Paramax. Analgesic/anti-emetic for migraine. **Metoclopramide** aids drug absorption by relief of the gastric stasis which can occur during a migraine attack as well as acting as an anti-emetic: see **Metoclopramide, Paracetamol**.

Paramol. Analgesic: see **Co-dydramol**.

Paramol-118. Analgesic: see **Dihydrocodeine, Paracetamol**.

Pardale. Analgesic/antipyretic: see **Caffeine, Codeine, Paracetamol**.

Parentrovite. High-potency parenteral vitamins for treatment of alcohol or drug-induced psychosis and other debilitated conditions: see **Aneurine, Nicotinamide, Pyridoxine, Riboflavine, Vitamin C**.

Parfenac. Non-steroid anti-inflammatory cream: see **Bufexamac**.

Parlodel. Dopamine agonist: see **Bromocriptine**.

Parmid. Antiemetic: see **Metoclopramide**.

Parnate. Antidepressant monoamine oxidase inhibitor: see **Tranylcypromine**.

Paroven. Vitamin derivative for symptomatic treatment of aching associated with varicose veins: see **Troxerutin**.

Parstelin. Antidepressant monoamine oxidase inhibitor/tranquillizer: see **Tranylcypromine, Trifluoperazine**.

Parvolex. Injection for treatment of paracetamol overdosage: see **Acetylcysteine**.

Pavacol. Cough suppressant: see **Papaverine, Pholcodeine**.

Pavulon. Muscle relaxant: see **Pancuronium**.

Paxadon. Vitamin: see **Pyridoxine**.

Paxane. Hypnotic: see **Flurazepam**.

Paxidal. Anxiolytic/analgesic: see **Caffeine, Meprobamate, Paracetamol**.

Paxofen. Non-steroid anti-inflammatory/analgesic: see **Ibuprofen**.

Paynocil. Analgesic: see **Acetylsalicylic acid**. formulated with **Glycine** to reduce gastric irritation.

Ped-El. Electrolytes and trace elements for parenteral nutrition.

Penbritin. Antibiotic: see **Ampicillin**.

Pendramine. Chelating agent: see **Penicillamine**.

Penidural. Antibiotic: see **Benzathine penicillin**.

Penotrane pessaries. Anti-infective for vaginal infections: see **Hydrargaphen**.

Pentostam. Antimony derivative: see **Stibogluconate sodium**.

Pentovis. Sex hormone for post-menopausal symptoms: see **Quinestradol**.

Pentoxylon (d). Antianginal: see **Penterythritol tetranitrate, Rauwolfia**.

Peptard. Anticholinergic for peptic ulcers and abdominal colic: see **Hyoscyamine**.

Peptavlon. Hormone injection for tests of gastric secretion: see **Pentagastrin**.
Percorten M Crystules. Adrenocorticosteroid depot injection for treatment of adrenal insufficiency: see **Deoxycortone**.
Percutol. Vasodilator gel for application to skin in prophylaxis of angina: see **Glyceryl trinitrate**.
Pergonal. Hormone: see **Menotrophin**.
Periactin. Serotonin antagonist for stimulation of appetite: see **Cyproheptadine**.
Peritrate. Antianginal: see **Pentaerythritol tetranitrate**.
Peritrate SA. As Peritrate but in sustained-release formulation.
Pernivit. Vitamins for chilblains: see **Acetomenaphthone, Nicotinic acid**.
Pernomol. Topical treatment for chilblains: see **Camphor, Chlorbutol, Phenol, Soap spirit, Tannic acid**.
Peroidin. For hyperthyroidism: see **Potassium perchlorate**.
Persantin. For ischaemic heart disease: see **Dipyridamole**.
Pertofran. Antidepressant: see **Desipramine**.
Pethilorfan (c) (d). Narcotic analgesic plus narcotic antagonist. Recommended as an analgesic where there is an obvious risk of respiratory depression (e.g., to the foetus during labour: see **Levallorphan, Pethidine**.
Petrolagar No. 1. Purgative: see **Liquid paraffin**.
Petrolagar No. 2. As Petrolagar No. 1 plus **Phenolphthalein**.
Pevaryl. Topical antifungal for skin infections: see **Econazole**.
Phanodorm (c). Hypnotic: see **Cyclobarbitone**.
Pharmalgen. Insect venom, prepared from bees or wasps for desensitization in allergic individuals.
Pharmorubicin. Cytotoxic: see **Epirubicin**.
Phasal. Sustained-release antimanic: see **Lithium salts**.
Phazyme. For flatulence and dyspepsia: see **Simethicone**.
Phenergan. Antihistamine for topical and systemic use: see **Promethazine**.
Phenergan Compound. Cough linctus/decongestant: see **Ipecacuanha, Potassium guaiacolsulphonate, Promethazine**.
Phensedyl. Cough linctus/decongestant: see **Codeine, Ephedrine, Promethazine**.
Phiso-Med. Anti-infective for cleansing skin/hair: see **Chlorhexidine**.
Pholcolix. Cough/cold mixture: see **Paracetamol, Phenylpropanolamine, Pholcodine**.
Pholcomed. Cough linctus: see **Papaverine, Pholcodine**.
Pholtex. Cough linctus/decongestant: see **Phenyltoloxamine, Pholcodine**.
Phortinea. Topical antifungal: see **Nitrophenol**.
Phosphate-Sandoz. Effervescent phosphate supplement for hyperparathyroidism and other bone disease.
Phospholine iodide. Preparations for open-angle glaucoma: see **Ecothiophate**.
Phyldrox (c). Bronchodilator/sedative: see **Ephedrine, Phenobarbitone, Theophylline**.
Phyllocontin. For asthma and cardiac failure: see **Aminophylline**.
Physeptone (c). Narcotic analgesic: see **Methadone**.

Phytex. Topical antifungal paint: see **Boric acid, Salicylic acid, Tannic acid**.
Phytocil. Topical antifungal cream and powder: see **Chlorophenoxyethanol, Phenoxypropanol, Salicylic acid**.
Pib/Pib plus. Aerosol bronchodilator: see **Atropine methonitrate, Isoprenaline**.
Picolax. Saline purgative: see **Magnesium citrate, Sodium picosulphate**.
Pimafucin. Topical antifungal for skin, vagina or lungs (by inhalation): see **Natamycin**.
Piportil depot. Long-acting tranquillizer injection: see **Pipothiazine**.
Pipril. Parenteral antibacterial: see **Piperacillin**.
Piptal. Anticholinergic for peptic ulcers: see **Pipenzolate**.
Piptalin. As Piptal plus **Simethicone** for abdominal colic.
Piriton. Antihistamine: see **Chlorpheniramine**.
Pitressin. Hormone: see **Vasopressin**.
P.K. Aid 1 (b). Dietary aid for phenylketonuria.
Plancaps. Haematinic: see **Ferrous Fumarate**.
Plaquenil. Anti-inflammatory: see **Hydroxychloroquine**.
Platinex. Cytotoxic: see **Cisplatin**.
Platosin. Cytotoxic: see **Cisplatin**.
Plesmet. For iron-deficiency anaemia: see **Ferrous sulphate**.
Plex-Hormone. Male sex hormone replacement: see **Deoxycortone, Ethinyloestradiol, Methyltestosterone, Vitamin E**.
Pneumovax. Vaccine for pneumococcal pneumonia.
Point-two. Mouth wash for prevention of dental caries: see **Sodium fluoride**.
Pollinex. Pollen extracts for desensitization in asthma, hay fever.
Polyalk. Antacid: see **Aluminium hydroxide, Dimethicone**.
Polybactrin. Antibiotic: see **Bacitracin, Neomycin, Polymyxin B**.
Polycal (b). Source of carbohydrate for kidney, liver, and various metabolic diseases.
Polycose (b). Lactose- and **Gluten**-free polysaccharide mixture.
Polycrol forte. Antacid: see **Aluminium hydroxide, Magnesium hydroxide, Simethicone**.
Polyfax. Antibiotic: see **Bacitracin, Polymyxin B**.
Polytar (b). Topical treatment for psoriasis: see **Coal tar**.
Polytrim. Antibacterial eye drops: see **Polymyxin B, Trimethoprim**.
Polyvite. Vitamin mixture: see **Aneurine, Calciferol, Nicotinamide, Pantothenic acid, Pyridoxine, Riboflavine, Vitamin A, Vitamin C**.
Ponderax. Anti-obesity: see **Fenfluramine**.
Pondocillin. Antibiotic: see **Pivampicillin**.
Ponoxylan. Topical anti-infective/anti-inflammatory: see **Polynoxylin**.
Ponstan. Anti-inflammatory/analgesic: see **Mefenamic acid**.
Portagen (b). Dietary aid for lactose intolerance.
Posalfilin. Topical treatment for warts: see **Podophyllum, Salicyclic acid**.
Potaba. Non-steroid anti-inflammatory: see **Potassium *para*-aminobenzoate**.

Pragmatar. Topical treatment for seborrhoea: see **Coal tar, Salicylic acid, Sulphur**.
Pramidex. Oral hypoglycaemic: see **Tolbutamide**.
Praminil. Antidepressant: see **Imipramine**.
Praxilene. Peripheral vasodilator: see **Naftidrofuryl**.
Precortisyl. Corticosteroid: see **Prednisolone**.
Predenema. Corticosteroid enema: see **Prednisolone**.
Prednesol. Corticosteroid: see **Prednisolone**.
Predsol. Corticosteroid: see **Prednisolone**.
Predsol-N. corticosteroid/antibiotic ear drops: see **Neomycin, Prednisolone**.
Prefil. Bulking agent, produces feeling of satiety and thus used to treat obesity: see **Guar gum, Sterculia**.
Prefrin. Eye drops for minor eye irritations: see **Phenylephrine**.
Pregaday. For anaemia of pregnancy: see **Ferrous fumarate, Folic acid**.
Pregestimil (b). Dietary aid for glucose, lactose, protein intolerance.
Pregfol (d). For anaemia of pregnancy: see **Ferrous sulphate, Folic acid**.
Pregnavite forte. For anaemia of pregnancy: see **Calciferol, Ferrous sulphate, Folic acid, Vitamin A, Vitamin B, Vitamin C**.
Pregnyl. Hormone: see **Gonadotrophin**.
Prehensol (d). Protective skin cream: see **Zinc salicylate**.
Premarin. Natural oestrogens from pregnant mare's urine for deficiency states.
Prempak. Sex hormones for replacement therapy at and after menopause: see **Norgestrel, Oestrogen**.
Pressimmune. Anti-human lymphocyte globulin for immunosuppression.
Pressurised Brovon. Bronchodilator aerosol: see **Adrenaline, Atropine methonitrate**.
Prestim. Antihypertensive: see **Bendrofluazide, Timolol**.
Priadel. Antidepressant: see **Lithium salts**.
Primalan. Antihistamine: see **Mequitazine**.
Primolut N. To reduce or postpone menstruation: see **Norethisterone**.
Primoteston depot. Male sex hormone for deficiency states: see **Testosterone**.
Primperan. Anti-emetic. Promotes gastric emptying: see **Metoclopramide**.
Prioderm. Topical treatment for lice: see **Malathion**.
Pripsen. For threadworms, roundworms: see **Piperazine**.
Pro-Actidil. Antihistamine: see **Triprolidine**.
Pro-Banthine. Anticholinergic used for antispasmodic and antacid effects: see **Propantheline**.
Procainamide Durules. Sustained release antidysrhythmic: see **Procainamide**.
Proctofibe. Non-digestible cellulose fibre similar to **Bran**.
Proctofoam HC. Topical treatment for ano-rectal conditions: see **Hydrocortisone, Pramoxine**.
Proctosedyl. Local treatment for haemorrhoids: see **Cinchocaine, Framycetin, Hydrocortisone**.
Prodexin. Antacid: see **Aluminium glycinate, Magnesium carbonate**.

Profasi. Hormone injection for use in certain forms of infertility and retarded sexual development: see **Chorionic gonadotrophin**.

Progesic. Non-steroid anti-inflammatory/analgesic: see **Fenoprofen**.

Progynova. Female sex hormone for deficiency states: see **Oestradiol**.

Proluton Depot. Hormone injection for prevention of habitual abortion: see **Hydroxyprogesterone**.

Prominal. Anticonvulsant: see **Methylphenobarbitone**.

Prondol. Antidepressant: see **Iprindole**.

Pronestyl. Antidysrhythmic: see **Procainamide**.

Propaderm. Topical corticosteroid: see **Beclomethasone**.

Propaderm A and C. Topical corticosteroid/anti-infective: see **Beclomethasone, Chlortetracycline, Clioquinol**.

Propain. Analgesic/antihistamine for headache and muscular pain: see **Caffeine, Codeine, Diphenhydramine, Paracetamol**.

Propine. Eye drops for chronic open-angle glaucoma: see **Dipivefvrin**.

Prosobee (b). Dietary aid for lactose intolerance.

Prosparol (b). Calorie source.

Prostigmin. Anticholinesterase: see **Neostigmine**.

Prostin E2. Prostaglandin: see **Dinoprostone**.

Prostin F2 Alpha. Prostaglandin: see **Dinoprost**.

Prostin VR. Prostaglandin: see **Alprostadil**.

Prothiaden. Antidepressant: see **Dothiepin**.

Pro-Vent. Sustained-release bronchodilator: see **Theophylline**.

Provera. For menstrual disorders and prevention of threatened abortion: see **Medroxyprogesterone**.

Provera 100 mg. High-dose **Medroxyprogesterone** for treatment of endometrial carcinoma or hypernephroma.

Pro-Viron. Male sex hormone for deficiency states: see **Mesterolone**.

P.R. Spray. Rubefacient: see **Chlorofluoromethane**.

Psoradrate. For treatment of psoriasis: see **Coal tar, Dithranol, Salicylic acid**.

Psorin. Ointment for topical treatment of psoriasis and eczema: see **Coal tar, Dithranol, Salicylic acid**.

Psoriderm preps. Topical treatments for psoriasis: see **Coal tar, Lecithin**.

Psoriderm-S. As Psoriderm plus **Salicylic acid**.

Psorigel. Topical solution for psoriasis: see **Coal tar**.

Pulmadil. Bronchodilator aerosol: see **Rimiterol**.

Pulmicort. Steroid aerosol for asthma: see **Budesonide**.

Pump-Hep. Anticoagulant for continuous infusion: see **Heparin**.

Puri-Nethol. Cytotoxic: see **Mercaptopurine**.

Pyopen. Antibiotic: see **Carbenicillin**.

Pyralvex. Topical anti-inflammatory for mouth ulcers: see **Anthraquinone glycosides, Salicylic acid**.

Pyridium. Analgesic for urinary tract: see **Phenazopyridine**.

Pyrogastrone. For oesophagitis due to gastric reflux: see **Aluminium hydroxide, Carbenoxolone, Magnesium trisilicate, Sodium bicarbonate**.

Q

Quellada. Topical treatment for scabies and lice: see **Gamma-benzene hexachloride**.
Questran. For hypercholesterolaemia: see **Cholestyramine**.
Quicksol. Purified crystalline beef insulin: see **Insulin**.
Quinaband. Impregnated bandage: see **Calamine, Clioquinol, Zinc oxide**.
Quinicardine. Antidysrhythmic: see **Quinidine**.
Quinocort. Anti-infective/corticosteroid cream for topical treatment of infected eczema and similar skin conditions: see **Hydrocortisone, Hydroxyquinoline**.
Quinoderm. Topical treatment for acne: see **Benzoyl peroxide, Hydroxyquinoline**.
Quinoderm with 1 percent hydrocortisone. As Quinoderm plus **Hydrocortisone**.
Quinoped. Topical antifungal for feet: see **Benzoyl peroxide, Hydroxyquinoline**.

R

Rabro. Antacid: see **Calcium carbonate, Frangula, Liquorice, Magnesium oxide**.
Ramodar. Non-steroid anti-inflammatory/analgesic: see **Etodolac**.
Rapifen (c). Narcotic analgesic: see **Alfentanil**.
Rapitard. Long-acting mixture of purified beef and pork insulins: see **Insulin**.
Rastinon. Hypoglycaemic: see **Tolbutamide**.
Rautrax. Antihypertensive: see **Hydroflumethiazide, Potassium chloride, Rauwolfia**.
Rauwiloid. Antihypertensive: see **Rauwolfia**.
Rauwiloid + Veriloid (d). Antihypertensive: see **Rauwolfia, Veratrum**.
Razoxin. Antitumour: see **Razoxane**.
RBC. Topical antihistamine: see **Antazoline, Calamine**.
Reactivan. CNS stimulant and vitamins for tonic: see **Aneurine, Cyanocobalamin, Fencamfamin, Pyridoxine, Vitamin C**.
Redeptin. Depot injection tranquillizers/anti-psychotic: see **Fluspirilene**.
Refolinon. Antagonizes antifolate cytotoxic drugs: see **Folinic acid**.
Regulan. Purgative: see **Ispaghula**.
Rehibin. For anovulatory infertility: see **Cyclofenil**.
Rehidrat. Electrolytes and sugars supplied in a powder for reconstitution into solution. Used orally to correct fluid and electrolyte imbalance (e.g., due to diarrhoea and vomiting).
Relaxit. Enema for constipation: see **Glycerol, Sodium citrate, Sodium lauryl sulphate, Sorbic acid**.

Relefact LH-RH. For diagnostic use in delayed sexual development and failure of pituitary gland function: see **Gonadorelin**.
Remnos. Hypnotic: see **Nitrazepam**.
Rendells. Spermicidal pessary/foam: see **Nonoxynol**.
Rescufolin. Antagonizes antifolate cytotoxic: see **Folinic acid**.
Resonium-A. Ion exchange resin: see **Sodium polystyrene sulphonate**.
Restandol. Male sex hormone: see **Testosterone**.
Retcin. Antibiotic: see **Erythromycin**.
Retin-A. Topical treatment for acne: see **Tretinoin**.
Rheumacin L.A. Sustained-release, non-steroid anti-inflammatory/analgesic: see **Indomethacin**.
Rheomacrodex. Plasma expander: see **Dextrans**.
Rheumox. Non-steroid anti-inflammatory: see **Azapropazone**.
Rhinamid (d). Nasal decongestant/anti-inflammatory: see **Butacaine, Ephedrine, Sulphanilamide**.
Rhinocort. Corticosteroid nasal spray for treatment of nasal symptoms, hay fever and other nasal allergies: see **Budesonide**.
Rifadin. Anti-tuberculosis: see **Rifampicin**.
Rifater. Anti-tuberculosis: see **Isoniazid, Pyrazinamide, Rifampicin**.
Rifinah. Anti-tuberculosis: see **Rifampicin, Isoniazid**.
Rikospray balsam. Aerosol spray for sore skin (e.g., nappy rash): see **Benzoin, Storax**.
Rikospray silicone. Aerosol spray for sore skin (e.g., bed sores): see **Cetylpyridinium, Dimethicone**.
Rimactane. Anti-tuberculosis: see **Rifampicin**.
Rimactazid. Anti-tuberculosis: see **Isoniazid, Rifampicin**.
Rimevax. Live attenuated **Measles vaccine** with **Neomycin** as antibiotic preservative.
Rimso-50. Used in bladder inflammation: see **Dimethyl sulphoxide**.
Rinurel. Analgesic/decongestant for symptomatic relief of the common cold: see **Paracetamol, Phenylpropanolamine, Phenyltoloxamine**.
Rite-Diet gluten-free (b). Dietary substitute for **Gluten** sensitivity.
Rite-Diet protein-free (b). Dietary substitute for protein intolerance (e.g., renal failure).
Rivotril. Anticonvulsant: see **Clonazepam**.
Roaccutane. Vitamin A derivative: see **Isotretinoin**.
Ro-A-Vit. **Vitamin A** supplement.
Robaxin. Muscle relaxant: see **Methocarbamol**.
Robaxisal forte. As Robaxin 750 plus **Acetylsalicylic acid**.
Robinul. Anticholinergic for peptic ulcers: see **Glycopyrronium**.
Robitussin A.C. Cough linctus: see **Codeine, Guaiphenesin, Pheniramine**.
Rocaltrol. Vitamin used for correction of calcium and phosphate metabolism in renal osteodystrophy: see **Calcitriol**.
Roccal. Skin antiseptic: see **Benzalkonium**.
Rogitine. For diagnostic test/treatment of phaeochromocytoma: see **Phentolamine**.
Rohypnol. Hypnotic: see **Flunitrazepam**.
Rondomycin (d). Antibiotic: see **Methacycline**.

Ronicol. Peripheral vasodilator: see **Nicotinyl tartrate**.
Ronyl. CNS stimulant: see **Pemoline**.
Rosoxacin. See **Acrosoxacin**.
Roscorbic. Vitamin: see **Vitamin C**.
Roter. Antacid: see **Bismuth subnitrate, Frangula, Magnesium carbonate, Sodium bicarbonate**.
Rotersept. Antiseptic spray for prevention of mastitis during lactation: see **Chlorhexidine**.
Rowachol. For biliary disorders: see **Camphor, Eucalyptus, Menthol**.
Rowatinex. For biliary disorders: mixture of **Essential oils** (e.g., **Anethole, Camphor, Eucalyptus**).
Rubelix. Cough linctus: see **Ephedrine, Pholcodine**.
Ruthmol. Salt substitute for low-sodium diets: see **Potassium chloride**.
Rybarvin. Bronchodilator aerosol: see **Adrenaline, Atropine methonitrate, Benzocaine**.
Rynacrom. Topical insufflation for allergic rhinitis: see **Sodium cromoglycate**.
Rythmodan. Antidysrhythmic: see **Disopyramide**.
Rythmodan retard. Sustained-release formulation of Rythmodan.

S

Sabidal SR. Sustained-release bronchodilator: see **Theophylline**.
Safapryn. Analgesic: see **Acetylsalicylic acid, Paracetamol**.
Safapryn-Co. As Safapryn plus **Codeine**.
Salactol. Topical treatment for warts: see **Lactic acid, Salicylic acid**.
Salazopyrin. For ulcerative colitis: see **Sulphasalazine**.
Salbulin. Sympathomimetic bronchodilator: see **Salbutamol**.
Saluric. Diuretic: see **Chlorothiazide**.
Salzone. Analgesic: see **Paracetamol**.
Sancos (d). Cough linctus: see **Menthol, Pholcodine**.
Sancos CO (d). Cough linctus/decongestant. As Sancos plus **Chlorpheniramine, Pseudoephedrine**.
Sandimmun. Immunosuppressant: see **Cyclosporin**.
Sandocal. Effervescent supplement for calcium deficiency states.
Sandoglobulin. Concentrate of **Immunoglobulin** for patients with deficiency of this protein.
Sando-K. Effervescent potassium supplement. Mixture of **Potassium chloride** and **Potassium bicarbonate**. Provides potassium and chloride ions for absorption. Gastric irritation much less than with simple potassium chloride solution. Some irritation may still occur. Danger of hyperkalaemia if used in renal failure, treated by haemodialysis and ion exchange resins.
Sanomigran. Migraine prophylactic: see **Pizotifen**.

Saventrine. Slow-release sympathomimetic for heart block: see **Isoprenaline**.
Savloclens. Disinfectant: see **Chlorhexidine**.
Savlodil. Antiseptic for skin wounds or burns: see **Cetrimide, Chlorhexidine**.
Savlon hospital concentrate. Antiseptic: see **Chlorhexidine**.
Schering PC4. Oral postcoital contraceptive: see **Ethinyloestradiol Norgestrel**.
Scheriproct. Topical treatment for haemorrhoids: see **Cinchocaine, Clemizole, Hexachlorphane, Prednisolone**.
Scoline. Muscle relaxant: see **Suxamethonium**.
SDV. Desensitizing vaccines for certain allergies (e.g., asthma).
Secaderm salve. Topical treatment for chilblains, boils, bunions: see **Phenol, Terebene, Turpentine oil**.
Secadrex. Antihypertensive: see **Acebutolol, Hydrochlorothiazide**.
Seconal sodium (c). Sedative/hypnotic: see **Quinalbarbitone**.
Sectral. Beta-adrenoceptor blocker: see **Acebutolol**.
Securon. Antianginal/antihypertensive: see **Verapamil**.
Securopen. Antibiotic: see **Azlocillin**.
Sedonan (d). Topical analgesic drops for painful ear infections: see **Chlorbutol, Phenazone**.
Selexid. Antibiotic: see **Pivmecillinam**.
Selexidin. Antibiotic: see **Mecillinam**.
Selora. Salt substitute: see **Potassium chloride**.
Selsun (b). Shampoo for seborrhoeic dermatitis: see **Selenium sulphide**.
Semi-Daonil. Oral hypoglycaemic: see **Glibenclamide**.
Semitard. Long-acting purified pork insulin (zinc suspension): see **Insulin**.
Senokot. Purgative: see **Senna**.
Seominal (c). Antihypertensive/sedative: see **Phenobarbitone, Reserpine, Theobromine**.
Septex No. 2. Antibacterial cream: see **Sulphathiazole, Zinc oxide**.
Septrin. Antibacterial: see **Co-trimoxazole**.
Serc. For Ménière's syndrome: see **Betahistine**.
Serenace. Tranquillizer: see **Haloperidol**.
Serenid-D/Serenid-Forte. Anxiolytic: see **Oxazepam**.
Serophene. For treatment of female infertility: see **Clomiphene**.
Serpasil. Antihypertensive: see **Reserpine**.
Serpasil-Esidrex. Antihypertensive: see **Hydrochlorothiazide, Reserpine**.
SH 420. Sex hormone for inoperable carcinoma of the breast: see **Norethisterone**.
Sidros. Haematinic: see **Ferrous gluconate, Vitamin C**.
Silbephylline (d). Bronchodilator: see **Diprophylline**.
Silderm. Topical corticosteroid/anti-infective: see **Neomycin, Triamcinolone, Undecenoic acid**.
Siloxyl. Antacid: see **Aluminium hydroxide, Simethicone**.
Simplene. Eye drops for glaucoma: see **Adrenaline**.
Sinaxar. Muscle relaxant: see **Styramate**.

Sinemet preparations. Antiparkinsonian containing varying doses of **Levodopa** plus **Carbidopa**.
Sinequan. Anxiolytic/antidepressant: see **Doxepin**.
Sinthrome. Anticoagulant: see **Nicoumalone**.
Sintisone. Corticosteroid: see **Prednisolone**.
Siopel. Soothing, antiseptic cream for skin rashes: see **Cetrimide, Dimethicone**.
Skin testing solutions. Allergen extracts used in skin testing for allergies.
Slo-Indo. Anti-inflammatory analgesic: see **Indomethacin**.
Slophyllin. Sustained-release bronchodilator: see **Theophylline**.
Sloprolol. Sustained-release beta-adrenoceptor blocker: see **Propranolol**.
Slow-Fe. Slow-release haematinic: see **Ferrous sulphate**.
Slow-Fe folic. Slow-release haematinic as Slow-Fe plus **Folic Acid**.
Slow-K. Slow-release **Potassium chloride**.
Slow-Pren. Sustained-release antihypertensive: see **Oxprenolol**.
Slow Sodium. Slow-release **Sodium chloride**.
Slow-Trasicor. Antihypertensive. Sustained-release formulation of **Oxprenolol**.
Sno phenicol. Anti-infective eye drops: see **Chloramphenicol**.
Sno-Pilo. Miotic eye drops for glaucoma: see **Pilocarpine**.
Sno Tears. Lubricant eye drops for dry eyes: see **Polyvinyl alcohol**.
Sodium Amytal (c). Hypnotic/sedative: see **Amylobarbitone**.
Sofradex. Corticosteroid/anti-infective drops for use in eyes or ears: see **Dexamethasone, Framycetin, Gramicidin**.
Soframycin. Topical anti-infective: see **Framycetin, Gramicidin**.
Soframycin inj. and tabs. Antibiotic: see **Framycetin**.
Sofra-Tulle. Gauze dressing with antimicrobial: see **Framycetin**.
Solis. Anxiolytic: see **Diazepam**.
Solarcaine. Local anaesthetic cream: see **Benzocaine, Triclosan**.
Solivito. Vitamins for injection: see **Aneurine, Biotin, Cyanocobalamin, Folic acid, Nicotinamide, Pantothenic acid, Pyridoxine, Riboflavine, Vitamin C**.
Soliwax. Softens ear wax: see **Dioctyl sodium sulphosuccinate**.
Solpadeine. Soluble, effervescent analgesic: see **Caffeine, Codeine, Paracetamol**.
Solprin. Soluble analgesic: see **Acetylsalicylic acid**.
Solu-Cortef. Corticosteroid injection: see **Hydrocortisone**.
Solu-Medrone. Corticosteroid injection: see **Methylprednisolone**.
Solvazinc. Soluble zinc supplements for zinc-deficiency states: see **Zinc sulphate**.
Somatonorm. Hormone: see **Somatrem**.
Somnite. Hypnotic: see **Nitrazepam**.
Soneryl (c). Hypnotic/sedative: see **Butobarbitone**.
Sòni-Slo. Sustained-release antianginal: see **Isosorbide dinitrate**.
Sorbichew. Antianginal, chewable tablets: see **Isosorbide dinitrate**.
Sorbid SA. Sustained-release vasodilator for prophylaxis of angina: see **Isosorbide dinitrate**.
Sorbitrate. Antianginal chewable tablets: see **Isosorbide dinitrate**.

Sotacor. Beta-adrenoceptor blocker: see **Sotalol**.
Sotazide. Antihypertensive: see **Hydrochlorothiazide, Sotalol**.
Sparine. Tranquillizer/anti-emetic: see **Promazine**.
Spasmonal. Antispasmodic for gastro-intestinal or uterine spasm: see **Alverine**.
Spectraban (b). Topical application for protection of skin from ultraviolet light.
Spectralgen. Injections of purified grass pollen allergens for treatment of pollen allergies.
Spiretic. Diuretic: see **Spironolactone**.
Spiroctan. Diuretic: see **Spironolactone**.
Spiroctan M. Diuretic: see **Potassium canrenoate**.
Spirolone. Diuretic: see **Spironolactone**.
Spiroprop. Antihypertensive: see **Propranolol, Spironolactone**.
Sprilon. Soothing, protective skin cream: see **Dimethicone, Zinc oxide**.
Stabillin V-K. Antibiotic: see **Phenoxymethylpenicillin**.
Stafoxil. Antibiotic: see **Flucloxacillin**.
Staycept. Spermicidal jelly: see **Octoxynol**.
STD inj. Scleroses varicose veins: see **Sodium tetradecyl sulphate**.
Stelabid. For reducing gastric motility, secretion, anxiety: see **Isopropamide, Trifluoperazine**.
Stelazine. Tranquillizer: see **Trifluoperazine**.
Steribath. Disinfectant bath concentrate: see **Iodine, Nonoxynol**.
Stemetil. Tranquillizer/anti-emetic/antivertigo: see **Prochlorperazine**.
Sterogyl-15. For calcium disorders: see **Calciferol**.
Ster-Zac (b). Topical anti-infective: see **Hexachlorophane**.
Stesolid. Anticonvulsant: see **Diazepam**.
Stiedex. Corticosteroid cream for dermatitis: see **Desoxymethasone**.
Stiedex LPN. Corticosteroid/antibiotic cream for infected dermatitis: see **Desoxymethasone, Neomycin**.
Stomogel (b). Stomal deodorant gel: see **Benzalkonium, Chlorhexidine**.
Strepsils. Lozenges for minor oral infections: see **Amylmetacresol, Dichlorobenzyl alcohol**.
Streptase. Fibrinolytic: see **Streptokinase**.
Streptotriad. Antibiotic/antibacterial: see **Streptomycin, Sulphadiazine, Sulphadimidine, Sulphathiazole**.
Stromba. Anabolic steroid: see **Stanozolol**.
Stugeron. Anti-emetic/antivertigo: see **Cinnarizine**.
Sublimaze (c). Narcotic analgesic: see **Fentanyl**.
Sudafed. Decongestant: see **Pseudoephedrine**.
Sudocrem. Bland topical cream for bed sores, nappy rash, and burns: see **Benzylbenzoate, Lanolin, Zinc oxide**.
Suleo (b). Shampoo for head lice: see **Carbaryl**.
Suleo-M. Topical treatment for lice: see **Malathion**.
Sulfamylon. Anti-infective cream for burns: see **Mafenide**.
Sulfapred (d). Antibacterial/corticosteroid eyes drops: see **Prednisolone, Sulphacetamide**.
Sulfomyl. Antibacterial eye drops: see **Mafenide**.

Sulphamezathine. Antibacterial: see **Sulphadimidine**.
Sulphatriad. Antibacterial combination: see **Sulphadiazine, Sulphamerazine, Sulphathiazole**.
Sultrin vaginal preps. Local antibacterial combination: see **Sulphacetamide, Sulphanilamide, Sulphathiazole**.
Suprol. Non-steroid anti-inflammatory analgesic: see **Suprofen**.
Surbex T. For vitamin B and C deficiency: see **Aneurine, Nicotinamide, Pyridoxine, Riboflavine, Vitamin C**.
Surem. Hypnotic: see **Nitrazepam**.
Surgam. Non-steroid anti-inflammatory/analgesic: see **Tiaprofenic acid**.
Surmontil. Antidepressive: see **Trimipramine**.
Suscard buccal. Vasodilator tablets for buccal absorption: see **Glyceryl trinitrate**.
Sustac. Antianginal: see **Glyceryl trinitrate**.
Sustamycin. Antibiotic: see **Tetracycline**.
Sustanon. Male sex hormone for deficiency states or inoperable breast carcinoma: see **Testosterone**.
Sylopal. Antacid: see **Aluminium hydroxide, Dimethicone, Magnesium oxide**.
Symmetrel. Antiparkinsonian: see **Amantadine**.
Sympatol. Vasoconstrictor: see **Oxedrine**.
Synacthen. Synthetic corticotrophic injection: see **Tetracosactrin**.
Synadrin. Antianginal: see **Prenylamine**.
Synalar. Corticosteroid: see **Fluocinolone**.
Synalar C and N. Topical corticosteroid/anti-infective: see **Clioquinol, Fluocinolone, Neomycin**.
Synandone. Corticosteroid: see **Fluocinolone**.
Syndol. Analgesic: see **Caffeine, Codeine, Doxylamine, Paracetamol**.
Synergel. Antacid: see **Aluminium antacids**.
Synflex. Non-steroid anti-inflammatory/analgesic: see **Naproxen**.
Synkavit. For prothrombin deficiency: see **Menadiol**.
Synogist. Shampoo for dandruff.
Synphase. Oral contraceptive: see **Ethinyloestradiol, Norethisterone**.
Syntaris. Topical corticosteroid spray for nasal allergies: see **Flunisolide**.
Synthamin. **Amino acids** and electrolyte sources for intravenous feeding.
Syntocinon. Synthetic pituitary hormone: see **Oxytocin**.
Syntometrine. Contracts uterine muscle: see **Ergometrine, Oxytocin**.
Syntopressin. Synthetic pituitary hormone: see **Lypressin**.
Synuretic. Diuretic combination: see **Amiloride, Hydrochlorothiazide**.
Syraprim. Antimicrobial: see **Trimethoprim**.
Syrtussar (d). Cough linctus: see **Dextromethorphan, Pheniramine**.
Sytron. For iron-deficiency anaemia: see **Sodium iron edetate**.

T

Tachostyptan. Promotes clotting: see **Thromboplastin**.

Tachyrol. Vitamin D analogue: see **Dihydrotachysterol**.
Tagamet. Gastric histamine receptor blocker; reduces acid secretion: see **Cimetidine**.
Talpen. Antibiotic: see **Talampicillin**.
Tambocor. Antidysrhythmic: see **Flecainide**.
Tamofen. For treatment of anovular infertility and breast cancer: see **Tamoxifen**.
Tampovagan. Pessaries containing **Stilboestrol** or **Neomycin** for vaginal complaints.
Tancolin. Cough suppressant: see **Dextromethorphan**.
Tanderil. Anti-inflammatory: see **Oxyphenbutazone**.
Taractan. Tranquillizer: see **Chlorprothixene**.
Tarband. Zinc and **Coal tar** bandage for eczema.
Tarcortin. Corticosteroid cream: see **Coal tar, Hydrocortisone**.
Taumasthman. Bronchodilator: see **Atropine sulphate, Caffeine, Ephedrine, Phenazone, Theophylline**.
Tavegil. Antihistamine: see **Clemastine**.
Tears Naturale. Drops for dry eyes: see **Dextrans, Hypromellose**.
Tedral. Bronchodilator: see **Theophylline, Ephedrine**.
Teejel. Gel for application to gums in dental pain: see **Choline salicylate**.
Tegretol. Anticonvulsant: see **Carbamazepine**.
Temetex. Corticosteroid cream: see **Diflucortolone**.
Temgesic. Analgesic: see **Buprenorphine**.
Tempulin. Long-acting purified beef insulin (zinc suspension): see **Insulin**.
Tenavoid. Diuretic/tranquillizer for premenstrual syndrome: see **Bendrofluazide, Meprobamate**.
Tenoret-50. Antihypertensive: see **Atenolol, Chlorthalidone**.
Tenoretic. Antihypertensive combination identical to Tenoret-50 but double dose of both drugs.
Tenormin. Beta-adrenoceptor blocker: see **Atenolol**.
Tensilon. Diagnostic for myasthenia gravis: see **Edrophonium**.
Tensium. Anxiolytic: see **Diazepam**.
Tenuate (c). Anti-obesity: see **Diethylpropion**.
Tercoda. Cough suppressant: see **Codeine**.
Tercolix. Cough suppressant: see **Codeine**.
Teronac (c). Anti-obesity: see **Mazindol**.
Terpoin. Cough suppressant: see **Codeine**.
Terra-Cortril. Antibiotic/corticosteroid: see **Hydrocortisone, Oxytetracycline**.
Terramycin. Antibiotic: see **Oxytetracycline**.
Tertroxin. Thyroid hormone: see **Liothyronine**.
Testoral. Male sex hormone: see **Testosterone**.
Textoral Sublings. Sublingual tablets for hypogonadism: see **Testosterone**.
Tetmosol (b). Topical treatment for scabies: see **Monosulfiram**.
Tetrabid. Antibiotic: see **Tetracycline**.
Tetrachel. Antibiotic: see **Tetracycline**.
Tetralysal. Antibiotic: see **Lymecycline**.
Tetrex. Antibiotic: see **Tetracycline**.

T-Gel. Shampoo for psoriasis, dandruff, eczema: see **Coal tar**.
Thalamonal (c). Narcotic analgesic/tranquilizer combination: see **Droperidol, Fentanyl**.
Thalazole. Antibacterial: see **Phthalylsulphathiazole**.
Thean (d). Bronchodilator: see **Proxyphylline**.
Theocontin Continus. Sustained-release bronchodilator: see **Theophylline**.
Theodrox. Bronchodilator/antacid: see **Aminophylline, Aluminium hydroxide**.
Theo-dur. Sustained-release bronchodilator: see **Theophylline**.
Theograd. Bronchodilator: see **Theophylline**.
Theosol (d). Bronchodilator: see **Theophylline**.
Thephorin. Antihistamine: see **Phenindamine**.
Theraderm. Topical treatment for acne: see **Benzoyl peroxide**.
Thiaver (d). Antihypertensive combination: see **Thiazide, Veratrum**.
Thovaline. Skin protective: see **Zinc oxide**.
Thytropar. Used in diagnosis of thyroid deficiency: see **Thyrotrophin**.
Ticar. Antibiotic: see **Ticarcillin**.
Tiempe. Antibiotic: see **Trimethoprim**.
Tigason. Used to treat psoriasis: see **Etretinate**.
Tiglyssin. Antispasticity: see **Tigloidine**.
Tildiem. Antianginal: see **Diltiazem**.
Timodine. Antifungal/corticosteroid cream: see **Benzalkonium, Dimethicone, Hydrocortisone, Nystatin**.
Timoped. Topical antifungal cream: see **Tolnaftate, Triclosan**.
Timoptol. Eye drops for glaucoma: see **Timolol**.
Tinaderm M. Topical antifungal: see **Nystatin, Tolnaftate**.
Tineafax. Topical antifungal: see **Zinc naphthenate, Zinc undecenoate**.
Tinset. Antihistamine: see **Oxatomide**.
Titralac. Antacid: see **Calcium carbonate**.
Tixylix. Cough suppressant mixture: see **Phenylpropanolamine, Pholcodine, Promethazine**.
Tobralex. Antibiotic: see **Tobramycin**.
Tofranil. Antidepressant: see **Imipramine**.
Tolanase. Oral hypoglycaemic: see **Tolazamide**.
Tolectin. Non-steroid anti-inflammatory/analgesic: see **Tolmetin**.
Tolerzide. Antihypertensive: see **Hydrochlorothiazide, Sotalol**.
Tonivitan A & D syrup. 'Tonic': see **Calciferol, Ferric ammonium citrate, Vitamin A**.
Tonivitan B syrup. 'Tonic': see **Aneurine, Nicotinamide, Pyridoxine, Riboflavine**.
Tonivitan caps. Vitamins for deficiency states: see **Aneurine, Calciferol, Nicotinic acid, Vitamin A, Vitamin C**.
Tonocard. Antiarrhythmic: see **Tocainide**.
Topal. Antacid: see **Alginic acid, Aluminium hydroxide, Magnesium carbonate**.
Topiclens. For wound irrigation: see **Sodium chloride**.
Topicycline. Antibiotic for topical application in acne: see **Tetracycline**.
Topilar. Topical corticosteroid: see **Fluclorolone**.

Torecan. Anti-emetic/antivertigo: see **Thiethylperazine**.
Tosmilen. Eye drops for glaucoma: see **Demecarium**.
Totolin (d). Decongestant: see **Phenylpropanolamine**.
Tracrium. Muscle relaxant: see **Atracurium**.
Trancopal. Tranquillizer: see **Chlormezanone**.
Trancoprin. Analgesic/muscle relaxant: see **Acetysalicylic acid, Chlormezanone**.
Trandate. Antihypertensive: see **Labetalol**.
Transiderm-Nitro. Transdermal preparation for prophylactic treatment of angina pectoris whereby the drug is applied to the skin a self-adhesive patch: see **Glyceryl trinitrate**.
Transvasin. Rubefacient: see **Nicotinic acid, Salicylic acid**.
Tranxene. Tranquillizer: see **Clorazepate**.
Trasicor. Beta-adrenoceptor blocker: see **Oxprenolol**.
Trasidrex. Antihypertensive: see **Cyclopenthiazide, Oxprenolol**.
Trasylol. Used in acute pancreatitis: see **Aprotinin**.
Travasept. Disinfectant: see **Cetrimide, Chlorhexidine**.
Travasept 30. Topical disinfectant to be used undiluted for wound and skin disinfection: see **Cetrimide, Chlorhexidine**.
Travogyn. For treatment of vaginal infections: see **Isoconazole**.
Tremonil. Antitremor: see **Methixene**.
Trental. Peripheral vasodilator: see **Oxpentifylline**.
Treosulfan. Cytotoxic: see **Threitol dimethane sulphonate**.
Trevintix. Anti-tuberculosis: see **Prothionamide**.
TRH. Hormone: see **Protirelin**.
Tri-Adcortyl. Topical corticosteroid/antibiotic: see **Gramicidin, Neomycin, Nystatin, Triamcinolone**.
Tribiotic. Antibiotic spray for use on skin: see **Bacitracin, Neomycin, Polymyxin**.
Tridesilon. Topical corticosteroid: see **Desonide**.
Tridil. Antianginal, for injection: see **Glyceryl trinitrate**.
Trifyba. High-fibre laxative extract of **Wheat husk**.
Trilene. Anaesthetic gas: see **Trichloroethylene**.
Trilisate. Non-steroid anti-inflammatory/analgesic: see **Choline magnesium trisalicylate**.
Triludan. Antihistamine: see **Terfenadine**.
Trimogal. Antimicrobial: see **Trimethoprim**.
Trimopan. Antimicrobial: see **Trimethoprim**.
Trimovate. Topical corticosteroid/anti-infective: see **Clobetasone, Nystatin, Oxytetracycline**.
Trinordiol. Oral contraceptive: see **Ethinyloestradiol, Levonorgestrel**.
TriNovum. Oral contraceptive with three different strengths for use at different stages of the menstrual cycle: see **Ethinyloestradiol, Norethisterone**.
Triocos. Cough suppressant/decongestant: see **Chlorpheniramine, Pholcodine, Pseudoephedrine**.
Triogesic. Decongestant/analgesic: see **Paracetamol, Phenylpropanolamine**.

Triominic. Decongestant/antihistamine: see **Pheniramine, Phenylpropanolamine**.
Triopaed. Cough linctus for children: see **Pholcodine**.
Triostam. Used in schistosomiasis: see **Sodium antimonylgluconate**.
Triotussic (d). Decongestant/antihistamine/analgesic: see **Paracetamol, Pheniramine, Phenylpropanolamine**.
Triperidol. Antipsychotic: see **Trifluperidol**.
Triplopen. Sustained-action antibiotic: see **Benethamine penicillin, Benzylpenicillin, Procaine penicillin**.
Triptafen DA/Forte/Minor. Antidepressant/tranquillizer: see **Amitriptyline, Perphenazine**.
Trisequens. Female sex hormones for menopausal symptoms: see **Norethisterone, Oestradiol, Oestriol**.
Trivax. Triple vaccination against diphtheria, tetanus, and pertussis.
Trobicin. Long-acting, single-dose antibiotic for gonorrhoea: see **Spectinomycin**.
Tropium. Anxiolytic: see **Chlordiazepoxide**.
Tryptizol. Tricyclic antidepressant: see **Amitriptyline**.
Trypure Novo. Enzyme for topical use in wounds and cavities to hasten removal of blood clots and slough.
Tubarine. Muscle relaxant: see **Tubocurarine**.
Tuberculin Tine Test. Intradermal injection test for tuberculosis: see **Tuberculin**.
Tuinal (c). Hypnotic: see **Amylobarbitone, Quinalbarbitone**.
Tussifans. Cough linctus: see **Belladonna extract, Ipecacuanha, Potassium citrate, Squill**.
Tyrozets. Local anaesthetic throat lozenges: see **Benzocaine, Tyrothricin**.

U

Ubretid. Anticholinesterase: see **Distigmine**.
Ukidan. Fibrinolytic injection: see **Urokinase**.
Ultrabase. Bland, protective cream recommended for use when topical steroids are withdrawn: see **Liquid paraffin, Soft paraffin, Stearyl alcohol**.
Ultradil. Topical corticosteroid for eczema: see **Fluocortolone**.
Ultralanum. Topical corticosteroid/anti-infective: see **Clemizole, Fluocortolone, Hexachlorophane**.
Ultraproct. Local treatment for haemorrhoids: see **Cinchocaine, Clemizole, Fluocortolone, Hexachlorophane**.
Ultratard. Long-acting purified beef insulin (zinc suspension): see **Insulin**.
Unguentum. Protective cream for use on skin. May be used as vehicle for drugs.
Uniflu plus Gregovite C. For symptomatic treatment of common cold: see **Caffeine, Codeine, Diphenhydramine, Paracetamol, Phenylephrine, Vitamin C**.

Unigesic. Analgesic: see **Caffeine, Paracetamol**.
Unihep. Anticoagulant: see **Heparin**.
Unimycin. Antibiotic: see **Oxytetracycline**.
Unigest. Antacid: see **Aluminium hydroxide, Dimethicone**.
Uniparin. Anticoagulant for subcutaneous injection: see **Heparin**.
Uniphylin. Sustained-release bronchodilator: see **Theophylline**.
Uniprofen. Non-steroid anti-inflammatory/analgesic: see **Ibuprofen**.
Uniroid. Local treatment for haemorrhoids: see **Cinchocaine, Hydrocortisone, Neomycin, Polymix B**.
Unisomnia. Hypnotic: see **Nitrazepam**.
Unitrim. Antibiotic: see **Trimethoprim**.
Urantoin. Urinary antiseptic: see **Nitrofurantoin**.
Ureaphil. Diuretic for intravenous infusion: see **Urea**.
Uriben. Antibiotic: see **Nalidixic acid**.
Urispas. Anticholinergic antispasmodic for urinary tract colic: see **Flavoxate**.
Urizide. Diuretic: see **Bendrofluazide**.
Urolucosil (d). Urinary anti-infective: see **Sulphamethizole**.
Uromide. Antibacterial/analgesic for painful urinary tract infections: see **Phenazopyridine, Sulphacarbamide**.
Uromitexan. Used to prevent bladder toxicity resulting from cyclophosphamide treatment: see **Mesna, Cyclophosphamide**.
Uro-Tainer. Sterile solution for maintenance of urinary catheters: see **Chlorhexidine, Magnesium citrate, Mandelic acid, Sodium chloride**.
Ursofalk. Bile acid for dissolution of cholesterol gall stones: see **Ursodeoxycholic acid**.
Uticillin. Urinary anti-infective: see **Carfecillin**.
Utovlan. Hormone: see **Norethisterone**.
Uvistat (b). Topical applications for protection of skin from ultraviolet light: see **Mexenone**.

V

Vaginyl. Antimicrobial: see **Metronidazole**.
Valium. Anxiolytic: see **Diazepam**.
Vallergan. Antihistamine: see **Trimeprazine**.
Valoid. Antihistamine: see **Cyclizine**.
Valrelease. Sustained-release anxiolytic: see **Diazepam**.
Vamin. Amino acids and carbohydrate for intravenous nutrition.
Vanair. Topical treatment for acne: see **Benzoyl peroxide, Sulphur**.
Vancocin. Antibiotic: see **Vancomycin**.
Vansil. Antischistosomiasis: see **Oxamniquine**.
Variclene. Used to clean skin ulcers. Contains brilliant green, a mild antiseptic.
Varidase. Enzymes for topical use in the removal of fibrinous or blood clots: see **Streptodornase, Streptokinase**.

Varihesive. Impregnated bandage: see **Carmellose, Gelatin, Pectin**.
Vascardin. Antianginal: see **Isosorbide dinitrate**.
Vasocon A. Topical antihistamine/vasoconstrictor anti-allergic preparations: see **Antazoline, Naphazoline**.
Vasculit. Peripheral vasodilator: see **Bamethan**.
Vasogen. Soothing, protective cream for sore skin: see **Calamine, Dimethicone, Zinc oxide**.
Vasolastine. Enzymes of lipid metabolism for vascular disorders and disorders of fat metabolism.
Vasoxine. Vasoconstrictor: see **Methoxamine**.
V-Cil-K. Antibiotic: see **Phenoxymethylpenicillin**.
Veganin. Analgesic: see **Acetylsalicylic acid, Codeine, Paracetamol**.
Velbe. Cytotoxic: see **Vinblastine**.
Velosef. Antibiotic: see **Cephradine**.
Velosulin. Purified crystalline pork insulin: see **Insulin**.
Ventide. Sympathomimetic/steroid aerosol for asthma: see **Beclomethasone, Salbutamol**.
Ventolin. Sympathomimetic bronchodilator: see **Salbutamol**.
Vepesid. Cytotoxic: see **Etoposide**.
Veractil. Antipsychotic: see **Methotrimeprazine**.
Veracur. Topical treatment for warts: see **Formaldehyde**.
Verdiviton elixir. Vitamin mixture: see **Aneurine, Cyanocobalamin, Nicotinamide, Pantothenic acid, Pyridoxine, Riboflavine**.
Veriloid (d). Antihypertensive: see **Rauwolfia**.
Veripaque. Laxative: see **Oxyphenisatin**.
Verkade (b). **Gluten**-free biscuits for gluten-sensitive bowel disorders.
Vermox. For threadworms, whipworms, roundworms, hookworms: see **Mebendazole**.
Verrugon. Ointment for warts: see **Salicylic acid**.
Vertigon Spansule. Sustained-release anti-emetic: see **Prochlorperazine**.
Verucasep. For treatment of warts: see **Gluteraldehyde**.
Vibramycin. Antibiotic: see **Doxycycline**.
Vibramycin-D. Water-dispersable antibiotic tablets, avoids the danger of oesophageal damage which may occur with capsules: see **Doxycycline**.
Vibrocil. Nasal decongestant/antibiotic: see **Dimethindene, Neomycin, Phenylephrine**.
Vi-Daylin. Vitamin mixture: see **Aneurine, Nicotinamide, Pyridoxine, Riboflavine, Vitamin A, Vitamin C, Vitamin D**.
Videne. Disinfectant: see **Providone-iodine**.
Vidopen. Antibiotic: see **Ampicillin**.
Vigranon B. Vitamin syrup: see **Aneurine, Nicotinamide, Panthenol, Pyridoxine, Riboflavine**.
Villescon. 'Tonic': see **Aneurine, Nicotinamide, Prolintane, Pyridoxine, Riboflavine, Vitamin C**.
Vioform-C. Topical anti-infective: see **Clioquinol**.
Vira-A. Antiviral ointment for eye infections: see **Vidarabine**.
Virormone. Hormone injection: see **Testosterone**.
Visclair. Reduces mucous viscosity: see **Methylcysteine**.

Viscopaste. Impregnated bandage: see **Zinc oxide**.
Vi-Siblin. Purgative: see **Ispaghula**.
Viskaldix. Antihypertensive: see **Clopamide, Pindolol**.
Visken. Beta-adrenoceptor blocker: see **Pindolol**.
Vista-Methasone N. corticosteroid/antibiotic nasal drops: see **Betamethasone, Neomycin**.
Vita-E. Vitamin: see **Vitamin E**.
Vitavel syrup. Vitamin mixture: see **Aneurine, Calciferol, Vitamin A, Vitamin C**.
Vitlipid. Fat-soluble vitamins for parenteral nutrition with fat solutions: see **Calciferol, Phytomenadione, Vitamin A**.
Vivalan. Antidepressant: see **Viloxazine**.
Vivonex (b). Dietary supplement of amino acids, glucose, fat, vitamins, and minerals.
Volital. CNS stimulant: see **Pemoline**.
Voltarol. Non-steroid anti-inflammatory/analgesic: see **Diclofenac**.

W

Wallachol. Oral preparations of vitamin B complex.
Waxsol. Drops to soften ear wax: see **Dioctyl sodium sulphosuccinate**.
Welldorm. Hypnotic: see **Dichloralphenazone**.
Wright's vaporizer. Inhalation for nasal, bronchial congestion: see **Chlorocresol**.

X

Xanax. Anxiolytic: see **Alprazolam**.
Xerumenex (d). Softens ear wax: see **Triethanolamine**.
X-Prep. Preradiography purgative: see **Senna**.
Xylocaine. Local anaesthetic: see **Lignocaine**.
Xylocard. Antiarrhythmic: see **Lignocaine**.
Xylodase. Topical local anaesthetic: see **Lignocaine**.
Xylomed. Used in the diagnosis of intestinal malabsorption: see **D-Xylose**.
Xyloproct. Local anaesthetic/corticosteroid for anal conditions: see **Hydrocortisone, Lignocaine**.
Xylotox preps. Local anaesthetic: see **Adrenaline, Lignocaine**.

Y

Yomesan. For tapeworms: see **Niclosamide**.
Yutopar. Uterine relaxant: see **Ritodrine**.

Z

Zactirin (d). Analgesic: see **Acetylsalicylic acid, Ethoheptazine**.
Zaditen. Antihistamine for prevention of asthma: see **Ketotifen**.
Zadstat. Anti-microbial: see **Metronidazole**.
Zantac. Gastric histamine receptor blocker. Reduces acid secretion: see **Ranitidine**.
Zarontin. Anti-epileptic: see **Ethosuximide**.
Zeasorb. Powder for excessive perspiration: see **Chloroxylenol**.
Zelmid (d). Antidepressant: see **Zimelidine**.
Zinacef. Antibiotic: see **Cefuroxime**.
Zinamide. Anti-tuberculosis: see **Pyrazinamide**.
Zincaband. Zinc paste bandage.
Zincfrin. Eye drops for conjunctival irritation: see **Phenylephrine, Zinc sulphate**.
Zincomed. For zinc deficiency: see **Zinc sulphate**.
Zomax (d). Non-steroid anti-inflammatory/analgesic: see **Zomepirac**.
Zonulysin. For cataract extraction: see **Chymotrypsin**.
Zovirax. Antiviral: see **Acyclovir**.
Z Span Spansule. Sustained-release zinc for zinc deficiency: see **Zinc sulphate**.
Zyloric. For gout: see **Allopurinol**.
Zymafluor. For prevention of dental caries: see **Sodium fluoride.**